THE
ATHLETE'S
PALATE®
COOKBOOK

THE
ATHLETE'S
PALATE®
COOKBOOK

**RENOWNED CHEFS, DELICIOUS DISHES,
AND THE ART OF FUELING UP WHILE EATING WELL**

YISHANE LEE AND THE EDITORS OF **RUNNER'S WORLD**®
FOREWORD BY MARK BITTMAN

RODALE®

© 2010 by Rodale Inc.

Rodale books may be purchased for business or promotional use or for special sales. For information, please write to: Special Markets Department, Rodale Inc., 733 Third Avenue, New York, NY 10017

Runner's World is a registered trademark of Rodale Inc.

Printed in the United States of America
Rodale Inc. makes every effort to use acid-free ♾, recycled paper ♺.

Photographs © Yunhee Kim
Additional photo credits: Page 11, © Sally Stein; Page 15, © Kate Sears; Page 27, © Rita Maas; Page 175, © Michael Lavine

"Penne Arrabbiata" and "Stir-Fried Beef with Scallions and Mushrooms" from *Get Saucy* by Grace Parisi, © 2005 by Grace Parisi. Used by permission of The Harvard Common Press.

"Kota Kapama" from *Cat Cora's Kitchen* by Cat Cora, Ann Krueger Spivak, and Maren Caruso, © 2004 by Catherine Cora. Used by permission of Chronicle Books.

"Curried Lentils with Butternut Squash" from *Cooking from the Hip* by Cat Cora and Ann Krueger Spivak, © 2007 by Catherine Cora. Used by permission of Houghton Mifflin Company.

Book design by Chris Rhoads

Library of Congress Cataloging-in-Publication Data is on file with the publisher.

ISBN 978–1–60529–578–7   paperback

Distributed to the trade by Macmillan

2 4 6 8 10 9 7 5 3 1   paperback

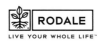

RODALE
LIVE YOUR WHOLE LIFE™

We inspire and enable people to improve their lives and the world around them
For more of our products visit **rodalestore.com** or call 800-848-4735

For every athlete who wants to eat well.

Contents

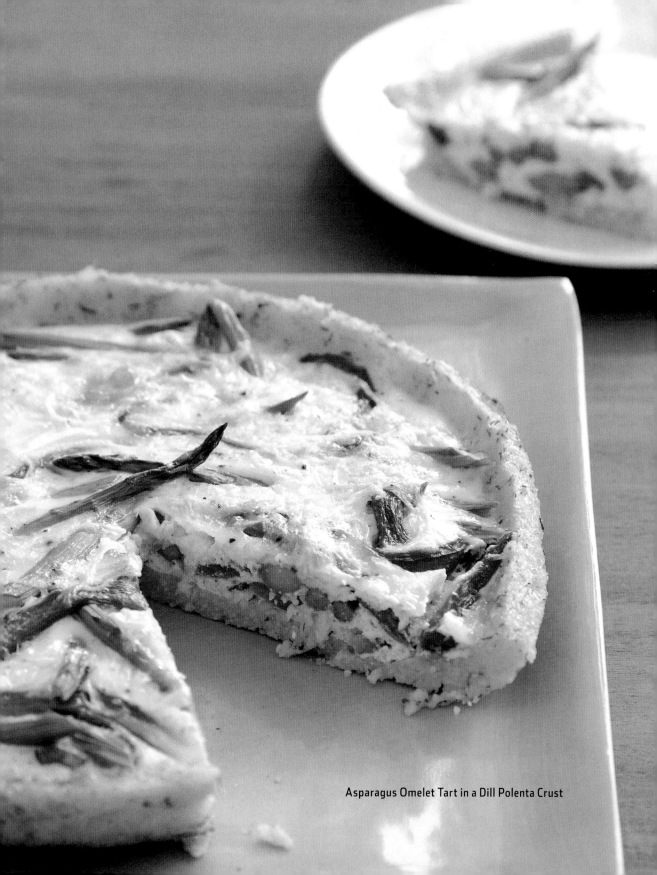

Asparagus Omelet Tart in a Dill Polenta Crust

Soups, Salads, and Sides

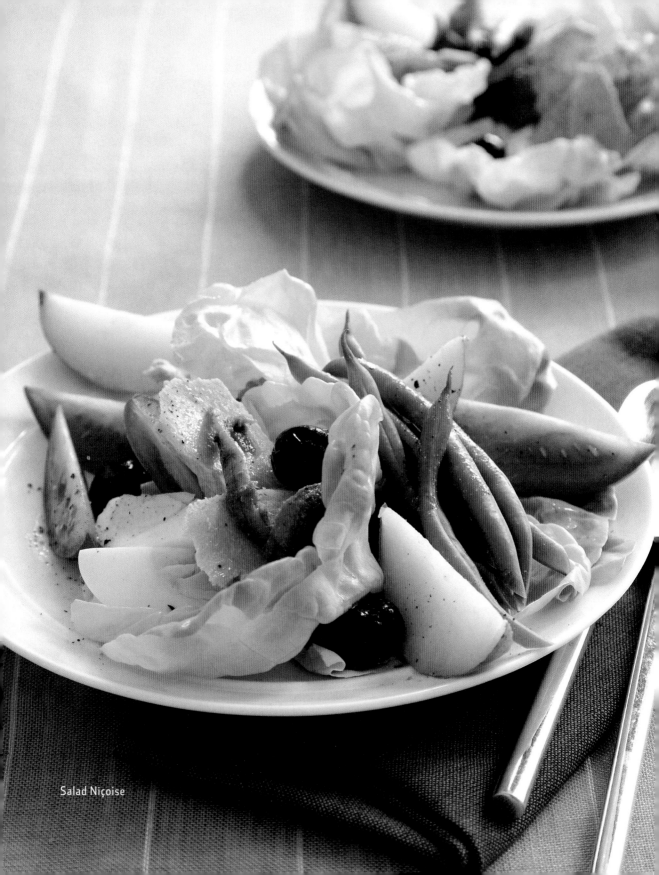

Salad Niçoise

Mains

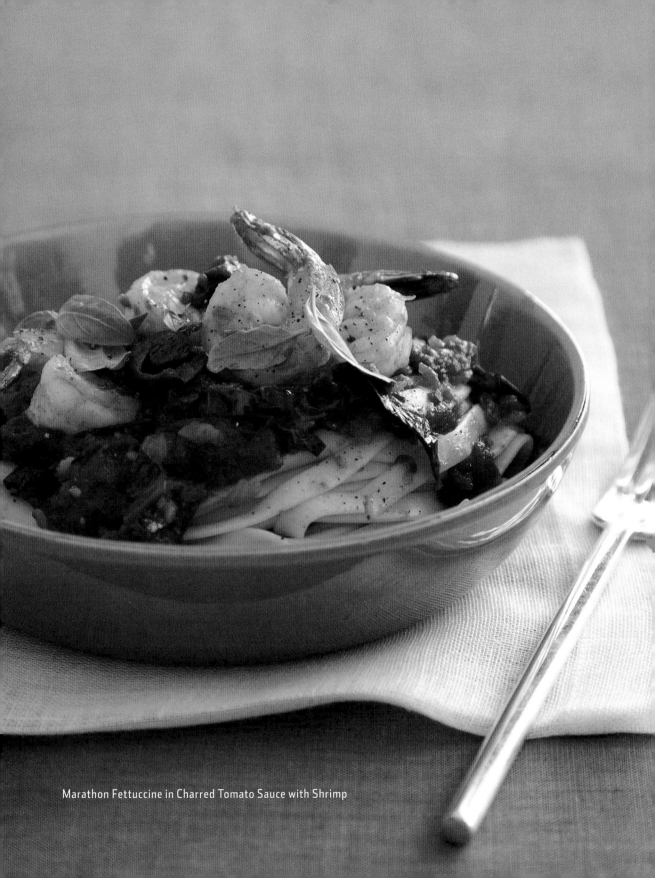

Marathon Fettuccine in Charred Tomato Sauce with Shrimp

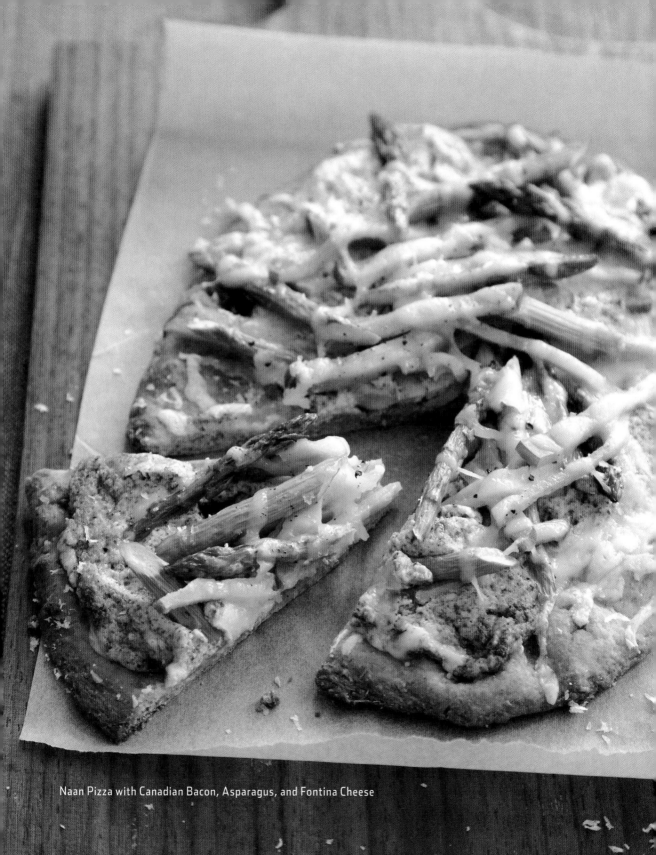

Naan Pizza with Canadian Bacon, Asparagus, and Fontina Cheese

Beverages

Desserts

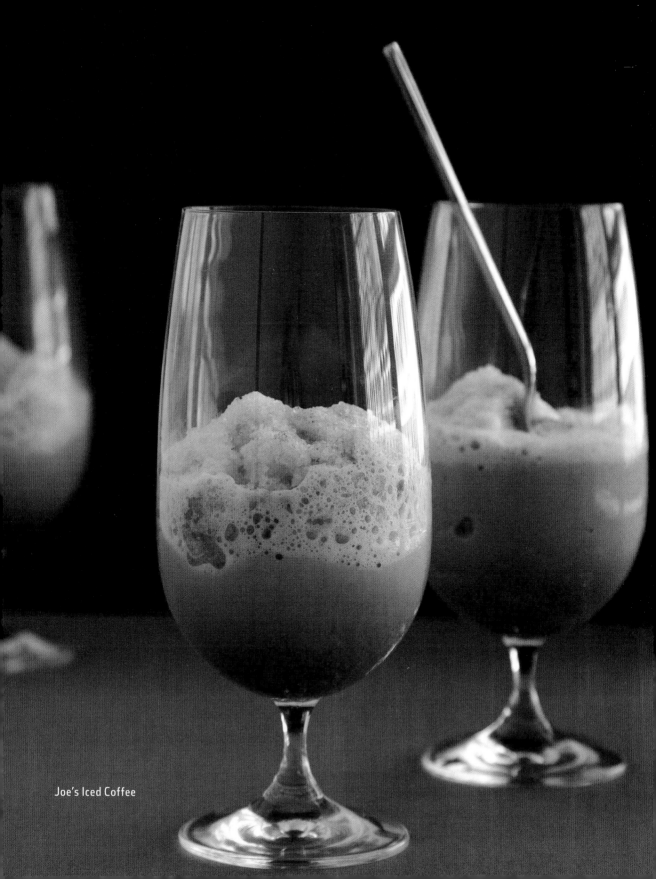

Joe's Iced Coffee

Foreword

I began cooking before I began running, so by the time I started pounding the pavement in 1976, there was always decent food in my house. But within a few years, my running and my cooking became much more serious. I started writing about food professionally in 1980. (I haven't yet managed to figure out how to run professionally.)

For me, running was part of a health kick. I decided to stop smoking in anticipation of the birth of my first daughter and thought running might help me quit. (It did.) Within a couple of years, 6- and 8-mile runs became routine and 10- and 12-mile runs weren't awe-inspiring.

Ten years later, I ran my first of five marathons. I finished the 1986 Stamford Classic Marathon in Connecticut in a satisfying 4:20. Of course, the post-long-run roaring hunger made me eat more—and, in my case, cook more. To me, running and cooking are both uncomplicated pleasures, enjoyed with minimum equipment and time.

Unintentionally, my career was built on this premise, and I've become known as someone who cooks "non-cheferly," straightforward food. I've always said that all you need is a few ingredients and a little time to produce great meals. For runners, this has special appeal, since we're often tired, usually busy, and always hungry.

That's where this cookbook can help. The chefs who have contributed to "The Athlete's Palate" column since its 2004 debut in *Runner's World* magazine are a diverse lot. Some have restaurants around the world or even appear on their own television shows, while others oversee neighborhood bakeries with devoted customers they know by name. They all have these important things in common: They love to cook, they love to exercise, and they love to eat.

The recipes they've contributed answer the question of what to eat before, after, and even during exercise. Whether a dish is simple and suited for a quick weeknight dinner or is a calorie splurge and company-worthy, the recipes give athletes a wealth of tasty options for every meal of the day, as well as for snacking and dessert.

Each contains nutritional benefits, but the point of the book is as much fueling for a race as it is enjoying the fuel itself. What follows are 100-plus delicious reasons to put on your running shoes, your swimsuit, your bike pedal clips, or your hiking boots and to simply enjoy eating, and eating well.

Mark Bittman is a contributing chef to *Runner's World* magazine's "Athlete's Palate" column. He is one of the country's best-known and widely admired food personalities and the author of a dozen books, including *How to Cook Everything* and *Food Matters*. He is also the creator of the popular cooking column in the *New York Times*, "The Minimalist," which debuted in September 1997.

—Mark Bittman

Introduction

Food is fuel, and no one is more keenly aware of this than athletes. Ask runners why they run, bicyclists why they bike, and triathletes why they do everything, and more often than not you'll get the answer "to eat, and to eat well." This cookbook celebrates eating well in every sense of the word—food that is good to eat and good for you.

When the editors of *Runner's World* magazine came up with the idea of "The Athlete's Palate" column, which debuted in 2004, the objective was to profile chefs who were also runners and to learn what their favorite dishes were for fueling and recovery. Running and cooking are both obsession-worthy activities, and it was never a challenge to find chefs who are as passionate about running as they are about cooking, whose four stars may be dwarfed only by their fastest time.

True, often chefs have notoriously poor habits when it comes to eating and exercise. They must taste dishes all day, and long hours in the kitchen translates into not a lot of time to work out. That's precisely why running in particular is so popular an activity for chefs. To run you don't need special equipment or a partner to play with, and you can do it virtually anywhere and anytime and as intensely or as easily as you like. For chefs who juggle meal preparation and late nights and who may have a spare hour only in the afternoon between lunch and dinner seatings or when the kitchen closes at midnight, running is the perfect sport.

Running is also one of the most efficient ways to burn calories. You burn four times as many net calories—that is, the total calories burned minus the calories you'd expend at rest—per hour than walking. And exercise of any sort gives you more energy, lifts the mood, and relieves stress.

Chefs who run are absolutely aware of the symbiotic relationship between eating well and keeping fit, between what you eat and how you feel. Healthy food doesn't necessarily mean a diet of denial. Instead, it can include menus rich in taste and flavor as well as nutrients. Low fat doesn't equal low taste, nor does high carb mean plain pasta.

When you're making the effort to keep fit, you'll find that your body naturally craves what it needs—not heavy, greasy foods but, rather, high-quality carbs, proteins, and (yes) fats. What these chefs have found and what you'll find, too, is that eating and exercise are intrinsically tied together—when one improves, so does the other.

We've taken some of the guesswork out of what foods and nutrients to look for while training and when recovering from a workout. Recipes marked "training" are good dishes to consider while training for a big race. While there is often a mix of both, they favor carbohydrates over protein. Those marked "recovery" are good for helping your muscles recover and to replenish nutrients expended through exercise, such as potassium. And for athletes whose idea of cooking might be opening a can of spaghetti sauce, we have used the label "quick and easy" to designate dishes that are simple and quick to make.

—Yishane Lee

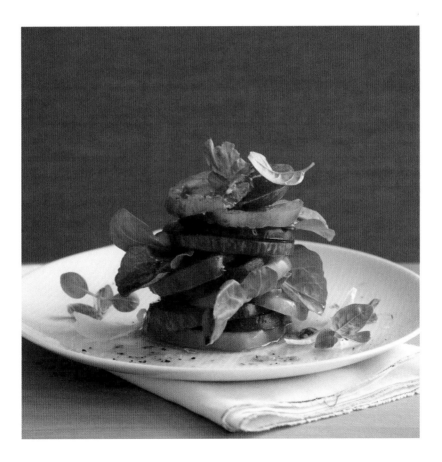

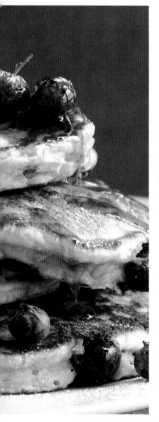

Breakfast

Not only is breakfast critical for refueling after a workout, it is also important for maintaining a healthy weight. Countless studies have shown that people who enjoy breakfast are better at managing their weight or even losing weight. Having a morning meal prevents you from becoming too hungry and prone to overeating later. And no wonder: Barring the midnight munchies, by the time the sun comes up your body has basically been fasting for up to 12 hours. Eating something in the morning will restore blood sugar levels—and put you in a better mood to face your workout and the day.

If you are moderately exercising early in the morning for an hour or less, a snack of 100 to 300 calories will be enough to power you through. This can be as simple as a glass of juice or a sports drink, gel, or bar. You can make your own using a recipe from Oregon chef Vitaly Paley, whose Energy Bar fuels with dried fruits and nuts.

Our running chefs' breakfast recipes will taste especially delicious when your workout is done. They provide quality protein and simple and complex carbs, along with some healthy fats. *New York Times* columnist Mark Bittman's Breakfast Couscous highlights a grain that fills you up without being too heavy. It's flavored with fruit and honey or maple syrup—all quick-energy sugars. Cookbook author Patricia Wells's Date and Walnut Bread is a dense quick bread filled with plenty of carbohydrates without too much fat. One added bonus: It packs well to bring to the starting line.

To get your fill of eggs, which many nutritionists consider the perfect protein, try New York City chef John Fraser's Spanish Tortilla or Pennsylvania chef Joe Carei's Asparagus Omelet Tart in a Dill Polenta Crust. And for traditionalists, "Iron Chef" Cat Cora's Walnut and Blueberry Bran Pancakes are a healthy update to a classic breakfast.

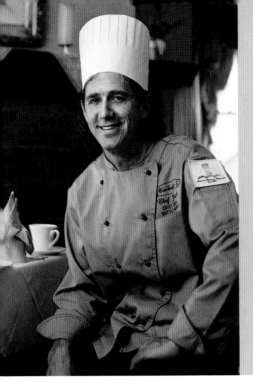

JOE CAREI

Like many runners, Joe Carei hits the road after work. Only as the chef-owner of two restaurants, he trades his clogs for trainers when the clock strikes midnight, when his workday ends. "It's a good way to take inventory of the day," says Carei, whose restaurants Caileigh's and Pasta Lorenzo are within a couple of miles of each other in Uniontown, Pennsylvania. In 2002, Carei launched Chef Joe's Omelet Run to benefit a 4-year-old with leukemia. The 5-K racers got omelets at the finish line, now an annual tradition. Yet at that inaugural race, the New Jersey native wasn't sure he'd see a second one. He, too, was battling cancer (of the colon), a struggle he says running helped him win. "Running goes through peaks and valleys," says Carei, who also hosts a local cable cooking show. "It helps you learn how to deal with life." For more, go to caileighs.com and pastalorenzo.com.

Asparagus Omelet Tart in a Dill Polenta Crust

RECOVERY

This omelet packs a nutritious punch. With 13 essential nutrients, the 75-calorie egg helps manage weight, strengthen muscles, and improve brain function and eye health. Asparagus is rich in folate and other B vitamins, as well as vitamins A, C, and K.

Makes 4 servings

PREP TIME: 20 MINUTES / BAKE TIME: 1 HOUR 20 MINUTES

Crust

3 cups reduced-sodium chicken broth

¾ cup coarse yellow cornmeal

1 tablespoon chopped fresh dill or 1 teaspoon dried dill

1 teaspoon freshly ground black pepper

(continued on page 4)

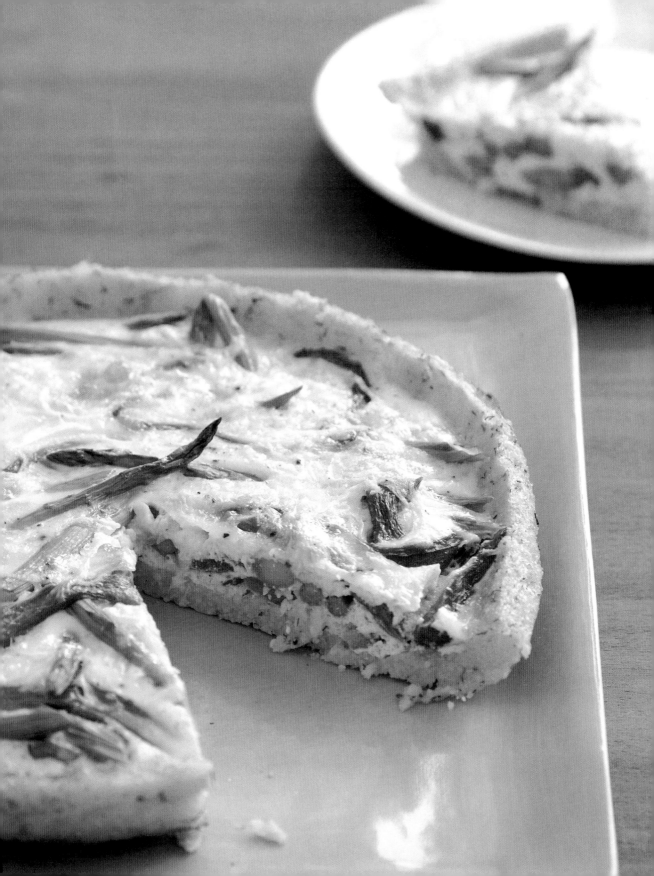

Filling

3/4 pound fresh asparagus, bottoms trimmed and cut into 2" pieces

1 roasted red bell pepper

4 large eggs

1/2 cup 1% milk

1/3 cup grated onion

1/2 teaspoon salt

1 teaspoon freshly ground black pepper

3/4 cup shredded fontina or Swiss cheese

3 tablespoons grated Parmesan cheese

Crust

Preheat the oven to 375°F. Bring the broth to a boil in a medium saucepan and whisk in the cornmeal slowly. Reduce the heat and simmer for 30 minutes. Stir frequently for 4 minutes, then mix every few minutes, always stirring in the same direction. When the polenta pulls away from the side of the pot, it's done. Add the dill and pepper, and mix. Spread the polenta evenly in a pie pan.

Filling

Blanch the asparagus for 3 minutes in boiling water. Cut the roasted pepper into strips. Whisk together the eggs and add the milk, onion, salt, and black pepper. Place the roasted pepper strips and asparagus in the bottom of the shell and top with the cheeses. Pour the egg mixture over the top and bake for 45 minutes.

PER SERVING: 299 CALORIES • 19 G PROTEIN • 26 G CARBOHYDRATES • 14 G FAT

BRIDGET BATSON

"After I quit smoking, I found that food tasted richer, sharper, and sweeter," says Bridget Batson. This certainly made her job as a chef easier. Swapping a 12-year-long cigarette habit for a running routine along San Francisco's Embarcadero, Batson shed 30 pounds in 8 months and is now a regular in San Francisco–area races, including the city's marathon and 12-K Bay to Breakers race. She also gained a new appreciation for her craft. "I wanted healthier ways to cook favorite foods, by relying on fresh, seasonal produce," she says.

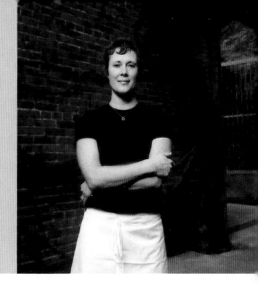

Quinoa Cookies

`QUICK AND EASY` `RECOVERY`

"Cookies made with quinoa flour instead of white flour get a nutritional boost," Bridget Batson says, "plus they have a nutty flavor." Because it contains nine essential amino acids, quinoa is considered a complete protein. Despite being considered a grain, it is actually a relative of spinach and chard. Find quinoa flour under the brand Bob's Mill at Amazon.com. You can also substitute all-purpose flour for the quinoa flour and cooked quinoa for the oats.

Makes about 2 dozen cookies

PREP TIME: 20 MINUTES + 20 MINUTES FREEZE TIME / BAKE TIME: 15–20 MINUTES

½ cup butter	½ cup quinoa flour
½ cup brown sugar	¼ teaspoon salt
½ teaspoon pure vanilla extract	½ teaspoon baking soda
1 egg, beaten	½ cup regular oats (not instant)
½ cup unbleached or all-purpose flour	½ cup fruit granola

Preheat the oven to 350°F. Cream the butter and brown sugar. Combine the vanilla and egg and add to the butter mixture. Sift the flours, salt, and baking soda and fold into the butter mixture. Fold in the oats and cereal.

Roll the dough into a log shape about 1½" to 2" in diameter using plastic wrap. Freeze for 20 minutes or until firm enough to slice. Slice into about 2 dozen ½" rounds. Place on a lightly greased baking sheet. Bake 15 to 20 minutes, or until crispy on the outside but still moist on the inside.

PER COOKIE: 100 CALORIES • 2 G PROTEIN • 12 G CARBOHYDRATES • 5 G FAT

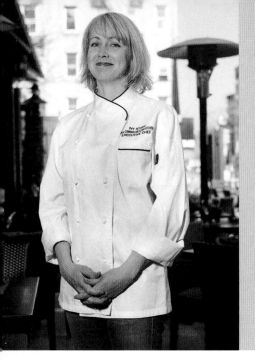

IVY STARK

A potato salad was Ivy Stark's "Eureka!" moment. "At age 6, I found it unbelievable that you could take such simple ingredients and make something so wonderful," says Stark, who is executive chef at New York City's Dos Caminos restaurant, which is known for its inventive Mexican cuisine. A state figure-skating champion in Colorado when she was a teenager, Stark says her experience in competitions helps in the kitchen. "The adrenaline rush I used to get out on the ice is the same rush I get now working as a chef," she says, "especially during a busy lunch or dinner service." Even routine 4-milers near her home in Brooklyn bring out her competitive spirit. "I feel like I'm running a race every day," she says. "New Yorkers are very competitive, even when they're relaxing." For more, go to ivystark.com.

Huevos a la Mexicana

QUICK AND EASY RECOVERY

Eggs are rich in protein, iron, and folate. The yolk is one of the best food sources for choline, a nutrient important for liver and cellular function, the metabolism of fat, and cardiovascular health. High choline levels are associated with better endurance and performance in runners. For more from Ivy Stark, see pages 76 and 114.

Makes 4 servings

PREP TIME: 15 MINUTES / COOK TIME: 10 MINUTES

2 tablespoons unsalted butter

½ medium white onion, finely chopped

2 serrano chili peppers, thinly sliced

2 plum tomatoes, washed and diced

6 eggs, beaten lightly with a fork

Salt to taste

1 bunch cilantro (about 1 cup), chopped

1 ripe avocado, peeled, seeded, and sliced

8 corn tortillas (8" diameter)

Melt the butter in a deep skillet, add the onion and chilies and cook, stirring frequently, until the onion is golden, about 5 minutes.

Add the tomatoes and the eggs, and cook until the eggs are done, about 5 minutes. Remove from heat.

Salt the eggs to taste. Warm the tortillas in a pan over low heat or in the microwave. Top the eggs with cilantro and avocado. Serve on a warm plate with warm tortillas on the side.

PER SERVING: 417 CALORIES • 17 G PROTEIN • 50 G CARBOHYDRATES • 17 G FAT

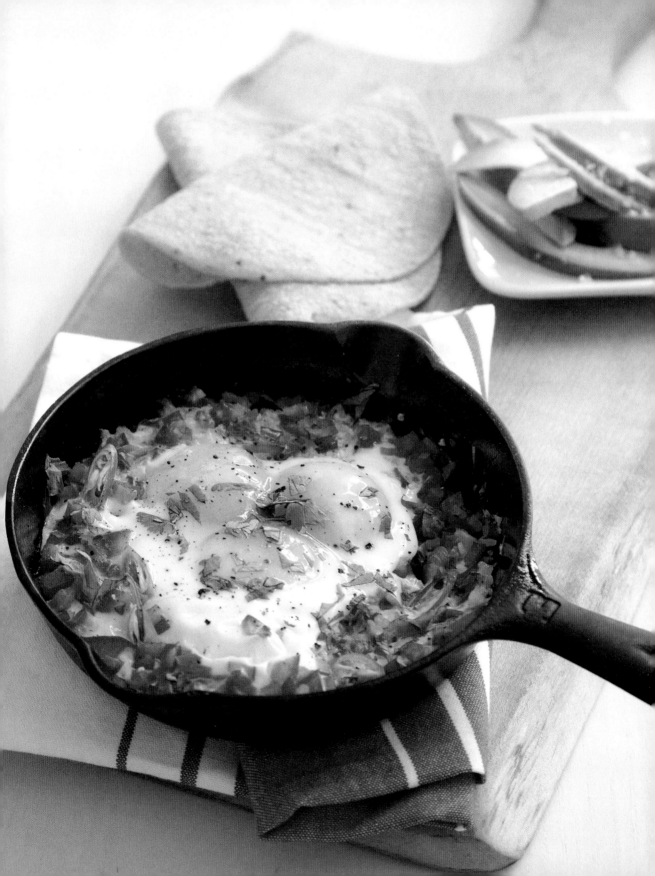

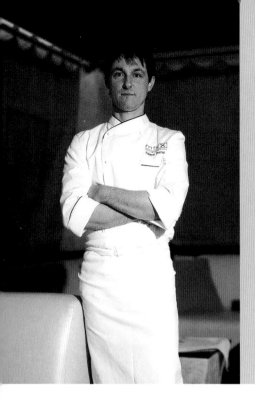

EDWYN FERRARI

A peripatetic career developing high-profile restaurants keeps Edwyn Ferrari on his feet. Good thing he's a triathlete, too, accustomed to making quick transitions among different sports. Having completed a couple dozen races, mainly sprint distance, Ferrari also snowboards, mountain bikes, and rock climbs, all activities suited to a recent stint advising restaurants in Colorado, where the New Jersey native settled briefly. Fresh from opening restaurants in and around New York City, many of them Asian-themed, Ferrari dipped into Mexican cuisine out west and also began studying ballet. "I wanted to get a stronger core and better balance to improve my climbing," Ferrari says. "Dance is by far the hardest thing I've done." Now back in New York City, he plans to continue studying modern dance and eventually open a sustainable-seafood restaurant.

Omelet Burrito

QUICK AND EASY / RECOVERY

Oaxaca cheese, also known as asadero, is a white cow's milk cheese that can be found in Spanish groceries or cheese specialty shops. "It tastes like something between mozzarella and unaged Monterey Jack," says Edwyn Ferrari, who suggests using Monterey Jack as a substitute. For more from Edwyn Ferrari, see page 141.

Makes 4 servings

PREP TIME: 15 MINUTES / COOK TIME: 10 MINUTES

1 teaspoon extra virgin olive or canola oil

1 clove garlic, chopped

1 small onion, thinly sliced

1 whole red or green bell pepper, thinly sliced

1 jalapeño chile pepper, seeded and sliced

2 plum tomatoes, chopped

Salt and ground pepper to taste

8 eggs

¼ cup 1% low-fat milk

1 cup Oaxaca cheese, grated

4 flour tortillas (10" diameter)

Heat the oil in a large skillet and cook the garlic, onion, bell pepper, and jalapeño over medium heat for 2 to 3 minutes, stirring frequently, until fragrant. Add the tomatoes and cook for an additional minute. Turn off the heat and season the vegetables with salt and pepper. Place the mixture in a bowl.

Whisk the eggs and milk together. Return the skillet to medium heat, and pour the egg mixture into the hot pan. Cook over medium heat, scrambling the egg mixture. When the eggs begin to set, add the sautéed vegetables and the cheese. Heat the tortillas in a separate pan over low heat or in the microwave until they are pliable, and divide the egg mixture among 4 tortillas. Fold the tortillas burrito-style and serve.

PER SERVING: 508 CALORIES • 27 G PROTEIN • 42 G CARBOHYDRATES • 26 G FAT

Spanish Tortilla with Greek Feta, Spinach, and Tomatoes

This Mediterranean casserole-style dish provides protein, iron, and calcium, thanks to the eggs, cheese, and spinach. Cooked tomatoes are rich in lycopene, which benefits eye health and can help prevent cancer and cardiovascular disease. For more from John Fraser, see page 80.

Makes 4 servings

PREP TIME: 10 MINUTES / COOK TIME: 50 MINUTES

2 medium Idaho potatoes, peeled

2–4 tablespoons extra virgin olive oil + more for coating the pan

8 eggs

½ cup Greek feta cheese, crumbled

1 cup baby spinach

1 cup diced tomatoes, fresh or canned

Salt to taste

Pinch of dried oregano

8 pitted kalamata olives, halved

Preheat the oven to 325°F. Use a mandoline to slice the potatoes into ⅓″ slices. Heat 2 tablespoons of oil in a medium-size skillet over low heat. Add the potato slices and cook, stirring frequently, for 10 minutes or until soft.

Coat a 9″ x 3″ loaf or terrine pan with oil.

Scramble the eggs in 2 tablespoons of olive oil in a saucepan and combine them with the potatoes, feta, spinach, tomatoes, 1 tablespoon olive oil, and a pinch of salt. Pour the mixture into a greased pan. Bake in the preheated oven for 35 to 40 minutes, or until a knife inserted comes out clean.

Sprinkle with the dried oregano and the olives.

Let it cool before slicing.

PER SERVING: 349 CALORIES • 18 G PROTEIN • 19 G CARBOHYDRATES • 23 G FAT

MARK BITTMAN

Mark Bittman started running when he stopped smoking, more than 3 decades ago. But by the time he turned 50, he admits, he had fallen into a common runners' trap: "I felt that I ran enough to compensate for overeating," he says. The author of more than a dozen cookbooks and books on food and a food columnist for the *New York Times* found that his career was becoming a hazard to his health. He had gained 40 pounds and found running 3 or 4 miles was a struggle. His cholesterol was high, he had sleep apnea, and his knees bothered him. "I couldn't run my way out of this one, so I decided to change my diet," Bittman says. He began eating more plants, fruits, whole grains, legumes, and nuts and fewer meats, processed foods, and junk food. The approach—as he details in his book *Food Matters,* which is subtitled "A Guide to Conscious Eating"—is better for the planet, and better for his health. In 2 months, he dropped 35 pounds, and his health has improved overall. After running five marathons in 10 years and then none for more than 10, he signed up to run the 2009 New York City Marathon. For more, go to markbittman.com.

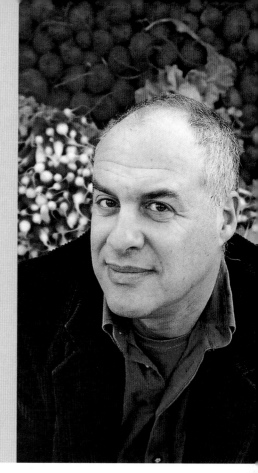

Breakfast Couscous

`TRAINING`

"Light, fast, easy to make, and in fact a complex carb, whole wheat couscous is one of my favorite prerun breakfasts," Mark Bittman says. He suggests making extra to eat as a side for dinner, since it reheats easily. For more from Mark Bittman, see page 26.

Makes 4 servings

PREP TIME: 10 MINUTES / COOK TIME: 10–20 MINUTES

1 cup whole wheat couscous (can substitute white)

1½ cups water

Pinch of salt

1 cup fresh fruit (sliced bananas, berries, diced apples, peaches)

¼ cup dried fruit, such as raisins, dates, or coconut (optional)

¼ cup chopped nuts (optional)

Drizzle of honey or maple syrup (optional)

(continued)

Put the couscous in a medium saucepan with a tight-fitting lid and add the water and a pinch of salt. Bring the water to a boil, then cover and remove from the heat. Let it steep for at least 10 minutes (5 minutes if using white couscous) or up to 20.

Add the fruit, nuts, and honey, if using. Fluff with a fork and serve.

PER SERVING (WITH BANANAS AND 1 TABLESPOON HONEY):
200 CALORIES • 4 G PROTEIN • 48 G CARBOHYDRATES • 1 G FAT

PER SERVING (WITH WALNUTS AND RAISINS):
280 CALORIES • 6 G PROTEIN • 57 G CARBOHYDRATES • 5 G FAT

Chocolate Cherry Muffins

David Chesarek suggests topping these muffins—which are good for breakfast, dessert, or a snack—with ready-made cream cheese frosting. Sweet cherries such as Bings contain vitamins C and A as well as calcium and iron. Antioxidant anthocyanins, which give cherries their red color, can reduce the inflammation that can come with exercise. For another recipe from David Chesarek, see page 165.

Makes 18 servings

PREP TIME: 20 MINUTES / BAKE TIME: 18 MINUTES

36–48 fresh cherries (about ¾ pound)

3 ounces cocoa

1 cup unbleached or all-purpose flour

1 teaspoon baking soda

¼ teaspoon baking powder

¼ teaspoon kosher salt

1 cup sugar

2 eggs

¾ cup canola oil

1 cup hot water

Preheat the oven to 325°F.

Line a cupcake tray with paper liners.

Pit and quarter the cherries, then set aside (48 cherries is roughly equal to 2 cups pitted and quartered).

Combine and sift the cocoa, flour, baking soda, baking powder, and salt, then set aside. Whisk together the sugar, eggs, and oil to combine. Whisk in the hot water.

Slowly add the dry ingredients to the wet ingredients and whisk together until combined. The batter will be slightly lumpy—don't overmix. Gently fold in the reserved cherries. Fill the liners about seven-eighths full with batter.

Bake for approximately 18 minutes, or until a toothpick inserted in the center comes out clean.

PER SERVING: 180 CALORIES • 3 G PROTEIN • 22 G CARBOHYDRATES • 11 G FAT

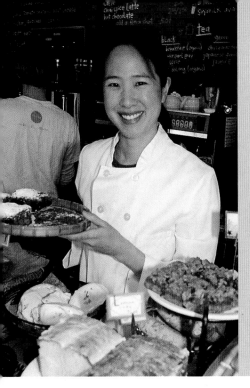

JOANNE CHANG

Before pastry chef Joanne Chang gets ready for a workout, she reaches for one of her own baked treats. "I end the workday with a cup of coffee and two pieces of banana bread for energy," says Chang, who oversees Boston's Flour Bakery and Cafe and, with her husband, the Chinese restaurant Myers + Chang. By the time Chang gets home from one of the bakery's two locations, she's ready for a 6-miler. The chef, who spent time in Texas as a child, stayed in Boston after graduating from Harvard with a degree in applied mathematics and economics. As a locally accepted bandit, she's raced the Boston Marathon every year from 1991 to 2006. "Even though I'm slower and slower, there I am at the start again," says Chang, who earned her best time of 4:15 her first year. "It's just impossible not to be swept up by the excitement." For more, go to flourbakery.com.

Flour's Famous Banana Bread TRAINING

This banana bread is a lightened version of a recipe that appears in Chang's cookbook, Flour. *Bananas provide potassium, which is important for balancing sodium and electrolyte levels and regulating blood pressure. The fruit is also a good source of fiber.*

Makes 12 servings

PREP TIME: 20 MINUTES **/** BAKE TIME: 45 MINUTES

$1^2/_3$ cups unbleached or all-purpose flour

1 teaspoon baking soda

$1/_4$ teaspoon ground cinnamon

$1/_2$ teaspoon salt

1 cup + 2 tablespoons sugar

2 eggs

$1/_4$ cup vegetable oil

$3^1/_2$ very ripe bananas, mashed

$1/_4$ cup unsweetened applesauce

2 tablespoons low-fat sour cream

1 teaspoon pure vanilla extract

$2/_3$ cup walnuts, toasted and chopped

Preheat the oven to 350°F. Butter a 9" x 4" loaf pan. Sift together the flour, baking soda, cinnamon, and salt and set aside. Beat the sugar and eggs with a whisk until light and fluffy. Drizzle in the oil. Add the bananas, applesauce, sour cream, and vanilla. Fold in the flour mixture and nuts. Pour into the prepared loaf pan and bake for 45 minutes, or until a toothpick inserted in the center comes out clean.

PER SERVING: 260 CALORIES • 4 G PROTEIN • 41 G CARBOHYDRATES • 9 G FAT

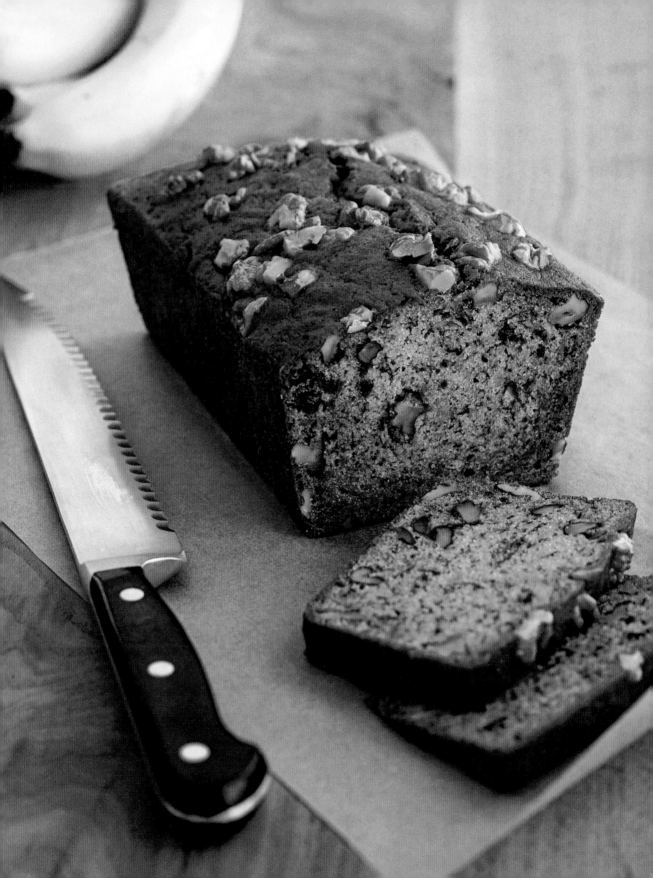

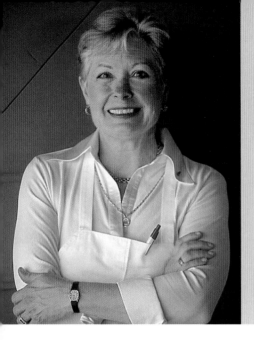

PATRICIA WELLS

A runner for more than 4 decades, Patricia Wells ran her first marathon on her 60th birthday in 2006. Since then, the France-based author of the upcoming *Salad as a Meal, Vegetable Harvest,* and 10 other books says she has been "racing like crazy." She ran the Paris Marathon and a handful of half-marathons, and each October she runs the 20 Kilometres de Paris, beginning and ending at the Eiffel Tower. "They give you timing chips you can keep, and each year the design is different," says Wells, a Milwaukee native who hosts a cooking school in Provence, France, and Paris. "I wear mine as 'charms' on my running shoes to remind myself that I can still do it." For more, go to patriciawells.com.

Date and Walnut Bread

TRAINING

Patricia Wells uses walnut oil in this carbohydrate-rich bread because "just a spoonful adds loads of flavor." The result is a dense, delicious quick bread that provides the energy a runner needs before a marathon. Plus, it can be easily packed into a race bag for a snack on the bus to the starting line, says Wells. For more from Patricia Wells, see pages 104, 181, and 194.

Makes 1 loaf

PREP TIME: 20 MINUTES / BAKE TIME: 40–50 MINUTES

1 teaspoon walnut oil	½ cup honey
1½ cups pitted and cubed dates	¾ cup hottest possible tap water
½ cup walnuts, toasted and coarsely chopped	2 large eggs, lightly beaten
½ teaspoon baking soda	1 teaspoon pure vanilla extract
½ teaspoon fine sea salt	1½ cups unbleached or all-purpose flour

Preheat the oven to 375°F. Coat a nonstick, 1-quart, rectangular bread pan with walnut oil. Set aside.

Combine the dates, walnuts, baking soda, salt, and honey in a large bowl. Add the hot water and stir to blend. Add the eggs and vanilla extract to the date mixture and blend thoroughly. Slowly add the flour and blend well. The batter will be fairly thick.

Pour the batter into the prepared pan, evening out the top with a spatula. Place the pan in the center of the oven and bake for 40 to 50 minutes, or until a toothpick inserted into the center of the bread comes out clean. Remove the bread from the pan and let it cool for at least an hour before slicing.

PER SERVING: 200 CALORIES • 3 G PROTEIN • 38 G CARBOHYDRATES • 4 G FAT

VITALY PALEY

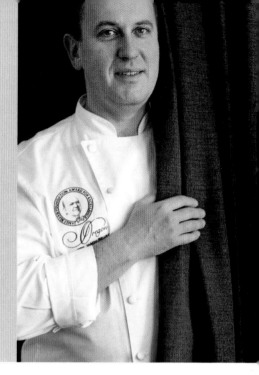

Vitaly Paley has a history of doing his own thing. The Russian native was a piano prodigy and left his country to attend Juilliard—then left Juilliard "to see what else was out there," he says. Paley went on to learn to cook in New York City and France. In 1995, he founded Paley's Place, a French-inspired restaurant in Portland, Oregon. So when the avid road cyclist couldn't find an energy bar he liked for his 60 to 80 weekly miles, he invented one. "I thought, *I'm a chef. I should be able to do this,*" Paley says of his namesake bars. The inspiration for one of the four PaleyBar flavors came from a favorite cycling route through berry fields on Sauvie Island north of the city. "You get whiffs of what smells like blackberry jam," he says. For more, go to paleysplace.net. For more from Vitaly Paley, see page 173.

Paley's Energy Bar

`QUICK AND EASY` `TRAINING`

An adaptation of the Fruity Nut PaleyBar, this energy bar is a good source of fiber and carbohydrates. Tart cherries are especially rich in the heart-protective antioxidants known as anthocyanins, which give cherries (and other red and blue fruits and vegetables) their color.

Makes 12 bars

PREP TIME: 20 MINUTES + REFRIGERATION TIME OVERNIGHT

¾ cup Turkish or Black Mission figs, stemmed and halved (about 3 medium fresh figs)

¼ cup raisins

¼ cup dried sour cherries

½ cup dry-roasted hazelnuts, chopped

2 tablespoons honey

2 tablespoons oat bran

Place the figs, raisins, cherries, hazelnuts, and honey in a food processor and pulse just until the batter comes together. Empty the batter onto a sheet of parchment or waxed paper. Sprinkle with the oat bran and press out the mixture with your hands until it is even in height all the way around, about ½" high and about a 9" x 12" rectangle. Wrap it tightly in plastic and let it firm up overnight in a refrigerator before cutting into 12 bars and serving.

PER SERVING: 64 CALORIES • 1 G PROTEIN • 10 G CARBOHYDRATES • 3 G FAT

Pink Grapefruit and Fig Tart

Pink grapefruit, like all citrus, is a great source of immunity-boosting vitamin C. One whole grapefruit provides more than 100 percent of your Daily Value. Its pink color comes from lyco- pene, an antioxidant also found in tomatoes that is associated with beating cancer and benefiting cardiovascular and eye health. Figs provide fiber and potassium, which helps regulates electrolyte and blood pressure levels. For another recipe from Jason Seraydarian, see page 51.

Makes 8 servings

PREP TIME: 45 MINUTES / BAKE TIME: 40 MINUTES

Shell

- ½ cup chopped pecans
- ½ cup whole wheat flour
- 1 tablespoon butter
- ¼ cup fresh dates
- 2 egg whites
- ¼ teaspoon salt

Filling

- 2 grapefruit, peeled and pith removed
- 1 whole cinnamon stick or ¼ teaspoon ground cinnamon
- 2 tablespoons honey
- 2 tablespoons sugar
- 2 cups fresh mission figs, halved (about 10 figs)
- 2 cups Greek-style yogurt

Shell

Preheat the oven to 350°F. Mix the pecans, flour, butter, and dates into a fine meal in a food processor. Add the egg whites and salt and process until fully incorporated.

Coat the inside of a tart pan with cooking spray. Line the bottom with a circle of parchment paper cut to fit, and coat again. Place the dough into the pan, and flatten it evenly with your fingers. There will be just enough dough to form a thin layer in the pan. Score the dough by poking it with a fork. Place a piece of parchment paper over the dough. Cover it with dried beans (this will hold the shell's shape, and you can use the beans again later), or use pastry weights. Bake the tart until the sides begin to brown, about 15 minutes. Remove the parchment paper and continue baking until the bottom has completely cooked, an additional 15 to 20 minutes.

The shell can be prepared in advance.

Filling

Cut out the grapefruit segments to use as a garnish, holding the fruit over a bowl to reserve the juice. You should yield about ½ to ¼ cup of juice, depending on the freshness of the fruit. Grate the peel of 1 grapefruit.

Place the cinnamon, honey, sugar, and reserved grapefruit juice together in a saucepan with the grated grapefruit peel. Allow it to simmer on low heat until the mixture begins to thicken, about 8 to 10 minutes. Remove it from the heat and allow it to cool. Once cooled, remove the cinnamon stick.

Mix together the figs, grapefruit segments, and the sweetened syrup in a bowl. Place 1 cup of yogurt in the bottom of the tart shell. Place the fruit mixture on top.

To serve, slice into portions and garnish with a dollop of the remaining yogurt.

PER SERVING: 240 CALORIES • 8 G PROTEIN • 39 G CARBOHYDRATES • 8 G FAT

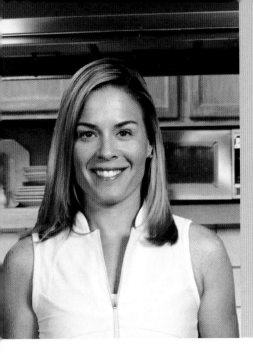

CAT CORA

These are the ingredients Cat Cora needs to be an "Iron Chef": a 7" Japanese knife, a mortar and pestle—and 45-minute running sessions three times a week. "It's sport cooking on the show," says Cora, who became the Food Network's first female Iron Chef in 2005. "I run around the whole time." No wonder Cora says her Pumas are one secret to her culinary success. A fan of yoga and cycling, too, the Santa Barbara–based chef and cookbook author believes in helping people understand that cooking isn't complicated or mysterious. She also established the nonprofit Chefs for Humanity to fight world hunger and increase nutritional awareness. "If you cook with flavor," Cora says, "then the nutrition will naturally follow." For more, go to catcoracooks.com.

Walnut and Blueberry Bran Pancakes `TRAINING`

Cat Cora uses whole milk, which health-conscious runners sometimes avoid, in her walnut and blueberry bran pancakes. "Fat is flavor," she says. "You just need a little bit to get the taste and to feel satisfied." For more from Cat Cora, see pages 120, 145, 155, 157, and 174.

Makes about 12 pancakes, or 4 servings

PREP TIME: 20 MINUTES / COOK TIME: 5 MINUTES PER PANCAKE

1½ cups whole milk

1 cup instant oats

¾ cup sifted unbleached or all-purpose flour (or a blend of white flour with oat flour or oat bran)

¼ cup oat flour or oat bran

¼ cup sugar

1 tablespoon baking powder

1 teaspoon salt

2 eggs, beaten

2 tablespoons honey

¾ cup fresh blueberries

½ cup chopped walnuts

Pour the milk over the oats in a large bowl. Lightly stir the eggs into the oats mixture. In a separate medium bowl, sift together the flour, sugar, baking powder, and salt. Add the sifted dry ingredients and the honey, stirring until combined. Gently fold in the blueberries and walnuts. Ladle the batter onto a preheated greased or nonstick griddle or skillet and cook until the tops are bubbly. Turn over and finish cooking the other side.

PER SERVING: 400 CALORIES • 15 G PROTEIN • 52 G CARBOHYDRATES • 16 G FAT

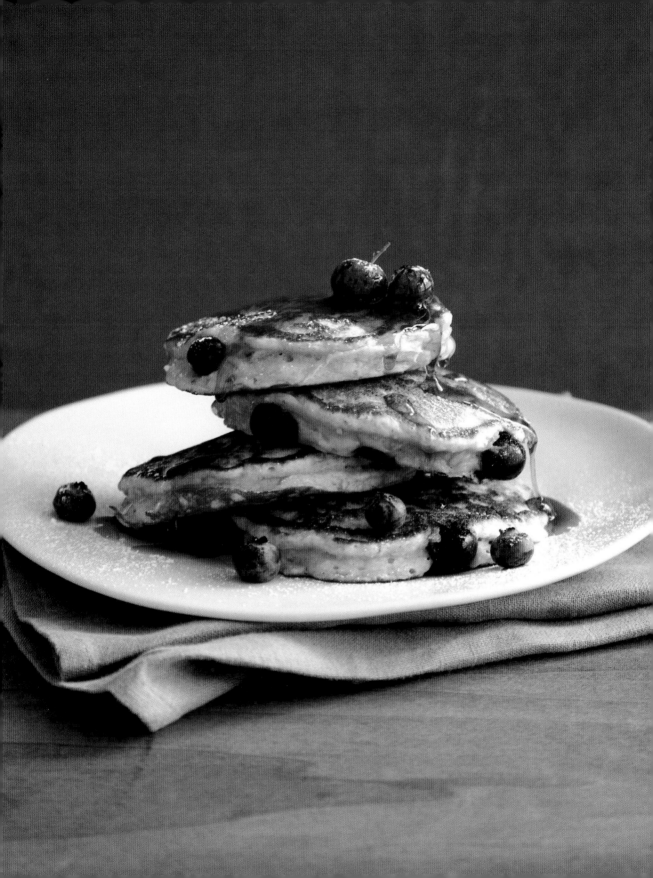

Power Breakfast Granola

Rolf Runkel likes this granola for breakfast or as a snack. "By mixing up the fruit you can create different variations," he says. "For instance, you can make a tropical granola with dried tropical fruits such as pineapple, papaya, and coconut." The ratio of nuts can also be increased or decreased, depending on your preference. "Once you make the first batch you won't even need a recipe anymore," Runkel says. "You can just do it by taste." For more from Rolf Runkel, see page 161.

Makes 6 cups

PREP TIME: 15 MINUTES PLUS 15 MINUTES COOL TIME / BAKE TIME: 15 MINUTES

2 cups old-fashioned rolled oats (do not use quick oats)

½ cup chopped walnuts or pecan

2 tablespoons flaxseed

2 tablespoons sunflower seeds (raw or roasted)

½ cup raisins

½ cup dried cranberries

¼ cup dried blueberries

½ cup chopped dried dates, prunes, dried apricots, or dried apples

½ cup dried banana chips (sweetened or unsweetened)

3 tablespoons honey

½ teaspoon cinnamon

½ teaspoon pure vanilla extract

Pinch of sea salt

Preheat the oven to 350°F. Place the oats, nuts, flaxseed, and sunflower seeds on a large cookie sheet and toast for 15 minutes, stirring once or twice to prevent burning.

Mix the raisins, cranberries, blueberries, dates, and banana chips in a large bowl.

Warm the honey and vanilla extract in a microwave oven. Stir in the cinnamon and salt.

Add the toasted oat mixture to the dried fruits, and mix until well combined. Pour the honey mixture over the oats and dried fruits and stir until the oats and fruits are slightly sticking. If you prefer a sweeter granola, just add more honey or a touch of brown sugar. Spread the mixture out on foil to cool completely, about 15 minutes.

Stored in an airtight container, the granola will keep for 10 to 14 days in a cool place. Do not refrigerate.

PER ½-CUP SERVING: 208 CALORIES • 4 G PROTEIN • 36 G CARBOHYDRATES • 6 G FAT

Zucchini Muffins

"This recipe is one of our and our customers' favorites," Beth Pilar says. "They are wonderful for breakfast or a quick snack." If you're not in the mood for muffins, bake the batter in a 9" x 5" loaf pan for 45 minutes to 1 hour. Eat it on its own or slice it for use in a sandwich. "The bread tastes great with turkey and cranberry sauce," Ellen Sternau says.

Shredded zucchini is an easy way to add both nutritional content and moisture to quick breads. It is an excellent source of vitamin C plus fiber, vitamin A, calcium, and iron, and contains only 20 calories per cup. Summer squash such as zucchini contains the phytochemical lutein, which promotes eye health. For more from Beth Pilar and Ellen Sternau, see pages 180 and 188.

Makes about 2 dozen muffins

PREP TIME: 20 MINUTES / COOK TIME: 25 MINUTES

2 cups unbleached or all-purpose flour

¾ cup granulated sugar

¾ cup light brown sugar

2 teaspoons baking soda

1 teaspoon baking powder

1 teaspoon ground cinnamon

1 teaspoon ground cloves

1 teaspoon ground nutmeg

1¼ cups vegetable oil

3 eggs

1 teaspoon pure vanilla extract

2 cups shredded zucchini (about 2 medium)

1 cup shredded carrot (about 1 large carrot)

1 cup coarsely chopped walnuts

1 cup mixed dried fruit such as currants, apricots, cherries

Preheat the oven to 325°F.

Combine the flour, granulated sugar, brown sugar, baking soda, baking powder, cinnamon, cloves, and nutmeg in a large mixing bowl. Mix the oil, eggs, and vanilla extract in another bowl, and pour into the dry mixture. Mix until thoroughly combined. Add the zucchini, carrot, walnuts, and dried fruit and mix until just combined.

Coat 2 muffin pans with cooking spray or line with paper liners.

Fill each muffin cup two-thirds full, using an ice cream scoop or a ¼-cup measuring cup. Place the pans on the center rack of the oven and bake for approximately 20 to 25 minutes, or until the muffins spring back when touched. Cool in the pan on a rack for 10 to 15 minutes. Remove from the pan and let the muffins cool completely directly on the rack.

PER SERVING: 246 CALORIES • 3 G PROTEIN • 27 G CARBOHYDRATES • 15 G FAT

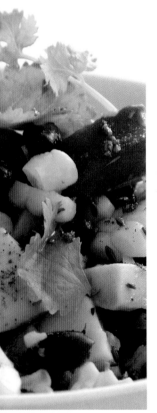

Soups, Salads, and Sides

Think of soups, salads, and sides as delicious ways to satisfy your appetite without filling you up too much. These dishes can act as preludes to the main event. Or, when you group several together tapas-style, they can be the main event itself.

On a hot summer's day, try Utah chef Christopher Sheehan's Shrimp and Artichoke Gazpacho. It's a twist on the traditional summer soup, replacing tomatoes with cucumbers for a refreshingly chilled dish. In wintertime, winemaker Andrew Murray's Sweet Butternut Squash Soup is a warming starter rich in potassium and beta-carotene.

For hearty soups that can double as entrées, try New York City chef Alex Raij's Lenten Chickpea Stew, cookbook author Pam Anderson's Hearty Ham and White Bean Soup, or Long Island chef Matt Connors's Ribollita. All three are stick-to-your-ribs fare, thanks to fiber-rich beans and vegetables.

Healthy and easy to prepare, salads are an athlete's best friend. Often they can become meals in themselves, as with San Francisco chef Thom Fox's Grilled Steak Salad. Poached egg adds a dose of protein to London chef Michel Roux's salad of endive and red onions.

But sometimes the simplest salads can be the most satisfying. Georgia chef Hugh Acheson's Tomato Salad is nothing more than heirloom tomatoes layered with arugula, basil, and cheese.

Cassoulet with Lots of Vegetables

Garbanzos de Vigilia
(Lenten Chickpea Stew)

Hearty Ham and White Bean Soup with
Cabbage and Carrots

Lentil and Kale Soup

Mango-Pear Soup with Ginger, Avocado and
Tomato

Potato Leek Soup with Steamed Clams

Ribollita

Shrimp and Artichoke Gazpacho

Succulent Potato Stew with Asparagus and
Shitake Mushrooms

Sweet Butternut Squash Soup

Arugula Salad

Baby Organic Field Greens with
Blood Oranges, Stilton Cheese, and Walnuts

Beef and Kombu Noodle Salad

Crab Salad with Avocado, Apple, and Green
Beans

Duck Breast and Beet Salad

Endive and Poached Egg Salad with Red
Onions and Dry-Cured Bacon

Kale Salad

Grilled Steak Salad

Roasted Corn Salad with Black Beans and
Avocado

Salad Niçoise

Salad of Port-Poached Figs with Point Reyes
Blue Cheese

Shaved Brussels Sprout Salad

Shrimp Noodle Salad

Spinach and Sweet Potato Salad with Bacon
Dressing

Tomato Salad

Warm Salad of Alaskan Halibut and Arugula

Baked Ricotta with Creamy Pesto Sauce

Cauliflower Flan

Grilled Spring Asparagus with Oven-Roasted
Tomato Salsa

Guacamole

Sizzle Fish

Cassoulet with Lots of Vegetables `RECOVERY`

Mark Bittman turns a classic on its head by transforming a meat dish laced with beans and seasoned with vegetables into a vegetable dish laced with beans and seasoned with meat. "There's plenty to satisfy everyone," he says. "You'll get the protein and bulk you're craving but without a lot of excess calories." For more recipes from Mark Bittman, see page 11.

Makes 4–6 servings

PREP TIME: 20 MINUTES / COOK TIME: 40 MINUTES

2 tablespoons extra virgin olive oil

1 pound skinless chicken legs (or Italian
   sausages, bone-in pork chops, confit duck
   legs, duck breasts, or a combination)

1 tablespoon chopped garlic

2 leeks or onions, trimmed, washed,
   and sliced

2 carrots, peeled and cut into 1" lengths

3 ribs celery, cut into ½" pieces

2 medium zucchini or 1 small head green
   cabbage, cut into ½" pieces

Salt and freshly ground black pepper
   to taste

4 cups chopped tomatoes, with juice
   (canned are fine)

¼ cup chopped fresh parsley

1 tablespoon chopped fresh thyme

2 bay leaves

4 cups cooked white beans or 2 (14 ounce)
   cans drained and liquid reserved

2 cups stock, dry red wine, bean cooking
   liquid, or water, + more as needed

⅛ teaspoon ground red pepper, or to taste

Heat the olive oil in a large saucepan over medium-high heat, add the meat, and cook, turning as needed, until the meat is deeply browned on all sides, about 10 minutes. Remove from the pan and drain off all but 2 tablespoons of the fat.

Reduce the heat to medium and add the garlic, leeks, carrots, celery, and zucchini. Sprinkle with the salt and pepper and cook until softened, about 5 minutes. Add the tomatoes, their liquid, the reserved meat, and the parsley, thyme, and bay leaves, and bring to a boil. Add the beans; bring to a boil again, stirring occasionally, then reduce the heat so the mixture bubbles gently but continuously. Cook for about 20 minutes, adding the liquid when the mixture gets thick and the vegetables are melting away.

Fish out the meat and remove the bones and skin as needed. Chop into chunks and return to the pot along with the ground red pepper. Cook 1 or 2 minutes longer to warm through, then taste and adjust seasoning if necessary and serve.

PER SERVING: 575 CALORIES • 40 G PROTEIN • 82 G CARBOHYDRATES • 11.5 G FAT

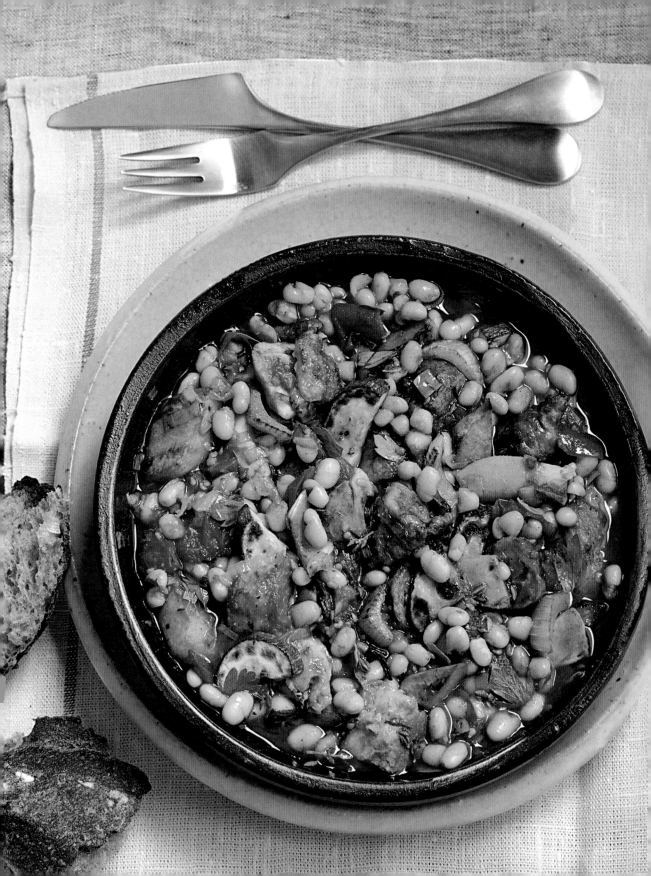

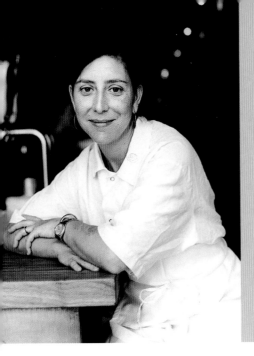

ALEX RAIJ

When Alex Raij was growing up in Minneapolis, she thought every kid ate tripe for dinner. "My parents are from Argentina, where meat is a big part of the diet," she says. "They threw big parties with pig roasts." Now at Txikito, a New York City restaurant that Raij owns, one signature dish is the trotters and tripe, a Basque specialty. The chef says running—a habit she picked up while trying to figure out what to do after college—taught her the discipline and inspires the creativity she needs in the kitchen. "I shop for produce at green markets, then drop off what I buy at the restaurant," says Raij, who logs about 20 miles a week. "Then I go for a run and think about how to incorporate what I bought." For more, go to txikitonyc.com.

Garbanzos de Vigilia (Lenten Chickpea Stew)

RECOVERY

"I like this dish because by using simple ingredients you can make something unique and healthy," Raij says. *Like most beans, chickpeas (garbanzos) are a great source of fiber, which helps clear out low-density lipoprotein (LDL or so-called "bad") cholesterol from the blood, as well as folate and magnesium, both beneficial for the cardiovascular system.*

Makes 8 servings

PREP TIME: 10 MINUTES + 24 HOURS TO REHYDRATE THE SALT COD / COOK TIME: 3 HOURS 30 MINUTES

1 pound dried chickpeas

1 Spanish onion, halved

1 unpeeled head of garlic + 3 cloves garlic, sliced thin

1 carrot

2 tablespoons + ¼ cup extra virgin olive oil

Salt to taste

1 tablespoon sweet paprika

2 pounds good-quality salt cod (bacalao), rehydrated per package directions and torn into small pieces, or substitute 2 pounds well-salted fresh cod (let rest for 10 minutes before rinsing)

6 cups fresh spinach leaves

Spanish olive oil (optional)

Cover the chickpeas with 8 cups of water in a large pot and bring to a boil. Remove the pot from the heat and let it stand at least 30 minutes to rehydrate.

Drain the chickpeas and return them to the same pot with the onion, head of garlic, and the carrot. Cover with 4″ of fresh water and add 2 tablespoons of the olive oil.

Partially cover the pot and bring it to a boil, then simmer the peas for 2 hours until they're tender, checking them frequently after the first hour and adding salt to taste. (Alternatively, you can cook them in a pressure cooker in about one-third of the time.) Remove the head of garlic and discard. Keep on low heat.

Heat the remaining $\frac{1}{4}$ cup olive oil in a small pan. Add the sliced garlic and stir until just golden. Pour the oil and garlic into a blender and add the paprika. Transfer $\frac{1}{2}$ cup of the rehydrated chickpeas, 1 cup of the cooking liquid, and the carrot and onion to the blender with the garlic and olive oil. Carefully blend the mixture to a smooth puree and add it back to the broth for body. (For a thicker stew, reduce the amount of water used and increase the amount of pureed chickpeas.)

Stir in the cod and spinach until cooked, about 5 to 7 minutes, or until the fish is opaque. Drizzle with olive oil and serve.

PER SERVING: 640 CALORIES • 83 G PROTEIN • 37 G CARBOHYDRATES • 16 G FAT

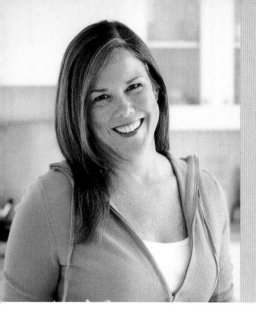

PAM ANDERSON

Cookbook author and former yo-yo dieter Pam Anderson knew something had to change when her weight hit a high of nearly 200 pounds in 2004. Instead of turning to another fad diet, she focused on eating healthy meals made with wholesome ingredients. She also started running daily—sometimes three two-milers a day—and in eight months dropped 45 pounds. Now Anderson, whose latest cookbook, *The Perfect Recipe for Losing Weight and Eating Great,* is a twice-yearly marathoner with seven 26.2's under her belt. For more, go to threemanycooks.com.

Hearty Ham and White Bean Soup with Cabbage and Carrots   QUICK AND EASY RECOVERY

This is a quick, hearty post-run soup," Pam Anderson says. To save time, microwave the chicken broth and tomatoes in a 2-quart Pyrex measuring cup while chopping the vegetables. For more from Pam Anderson, see pages 98 and 152.

Makes 3 quarts, or about 6 servings at 2 cups each

PREP TIME: 10 MINUTES / COOK TIME: 25 MINUTES

1 tablespoon extra-virgin olive oil

1 large sweet onion, chopped

1½ teaspoons Italian seasoning

2 large carrots, halved lengthwise and
    thinly sliced

½ small cabbage, cored and cut into bite-
    size shreds

12 ounces lean ham steak, finely diced

1 quart chicken broth

1 can (14.5 ounces) petite-diced tomatoes

2 cans (15–16 ounces each) white beans,
    undrained

2 tablespoons chopped fresh parsley
    (optional)

Heat the oil over medium-high heat in a soup kettle or a large pot. Add the onion and cook, stirring frequently, until soft and golden, about 5 minutes. Add the Italian seasoning and cook, stirring frequently, until fragrant, about 1 minute. Add the carrots, cabbage, ham steak, chicken broth, tomatoes, and beans. Bring to a full simmer. Reduce the heat to low and continue to simmer, partially covered, until the vegetables are just cooked, about 15 minutes. Stir in the parsley, if using. Cover and let stand for 5 minutes. Serve.

PER SERVING: 270 CALORIES • 22 G PROTEIN • 32 G CARBOHYDRATES • 6 G FAT

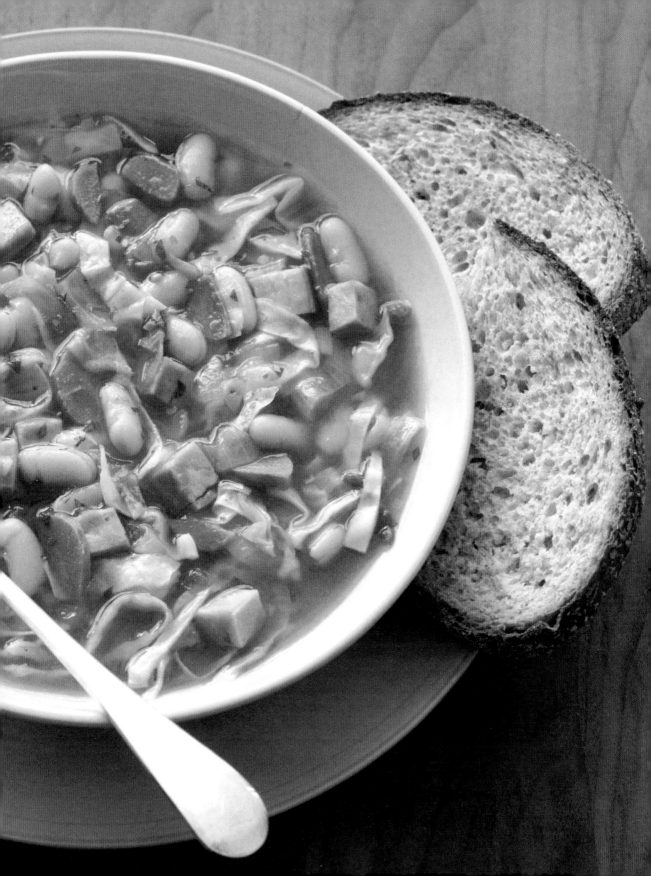

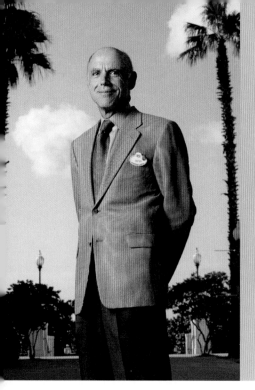

DIETER HANNIG

Visitors to Walt Disney World can thank Dieter Hannig for healthy food options at the theme park. His legacy as senior vice president of the resort's food and beverage division is gourmet food featuring locally grown, organic foods. While the park still serves its share of chicken nuggets and fries, you may also find such upscale entrées as lobster tail with mango chutney. "You really are what you eat," says Hannig, who is originally from Germany. "We wouldn't have an obesity problem if people focused on what they're putting into their mouths." The vegetarian is an accomplished athlete, rising at 4:30 a.m. to train for twice-yearly triathlons and the Disney Marathon, which he has completed a dozen times. Having departed the Magic Kingdom, Hannig has moved south to Panama where his next challenge is opening an organic food and yoga resort.

Lentil and Kale Soup

`TRAINING`

Petite green French lentils have a richer flavor than brown or red lentils. They also keep their shape and color, don't turn starchy in the mix, and are a good source of calcium, vitamins A and B, and iron.

Makes 6 servings

PREP TIME: 20 MINUTES / COOK TIME: 30 MINUTES

1 pound petite green French lentils

2 teaspoons sea or kosher salt

¼ cup extra-virgin olive oil + more for garnish

1 bay leaf

1 cup chopped onion

2 ribs celery, chopped

2 carrots, chopped

2 garlic cloves, mashed

1 large bunch kale, chopped (about 8 cups)

1 can (14.5 ounces) no-salt-added diced tomatoes

6 cups reduced-sodium, fat-free chicken broth

¼ cup fresh chopped parsley

¼ teaspoon freshly ground black pepper

Wash the lentils and place them in a soup pot. Cover them with water and add 1 teaspoon of the sea salt. Bring them to a boil and cook for 5 minutes. Drain and rinse. Heat the olive oil in the soup pot with the bay leaf, then add the onion, celery, carrots, and garlic and cook for 2 minutes. Add the kale and simmer for 5 minutes.

Stir in the tomatoes. Add the chicken broth, lentils, and the remaining sea salt. Blend all ingredients and bring to a boil. Reduce the heat and simmer for 15 to 20 minutes, until the lentils are tender. Add the chopped parsley and the ground black pepper.

Divide among 6 bowls and add freshly grated Parmesan cheese. Garnish with parsley and a few drops of olive oil before serving.

PER SERVING: 419 CALORIES • 24 G PROTEIN • 62 G CARBOHYDRATES • 10 G FAT

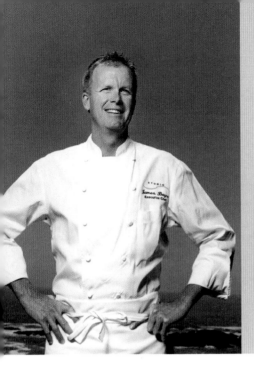

JAMES BOYCE

Years of long work hours, little exercise, and a poor diet took their toll on James Boyce's health. At 6'2", he weighed 300 pounds and ended up in the hospital after overexerting himself doing sports. "I was lying in bed, as big as a house," he says. "I realized everything that was wrong with me was self-inflicted." Boyce got serious about cutting calories and exercising. His favorite workout was to climb to the 2,704-foot summit of Arizona's Camelback Mountain, near where he lived at the time. Then he'd descend the mountain and run around the base. In a year he shed 120 pounds. Now he maintains a healthy weight with a regimen of running, yoga, cycling, and swimming while overseeing Cotton Row Restaurant in Huntsville, Alabama, and Pane e Vino at the Huntsville Museum of Art. For more, go to cottonrowrestaurant.com.

Mango-Pear Soup with Ginger, Avocado, and Tomato

QUICK AND EASY   RECOVERY

This cold mango-pear soup takes advantage of fruits at their peak in the summer months. Mangoes are very rich in vitamins A and C, while pears contain vitamin C and both fruits contain fiber. For more from James Boyce, see page 64.

For more from James Boyce, see page 64.

Makes 6 servings

PREP TIME: 20 MINUTES

2 very ripe mangoes, peeled and cored

2 very ripe pears, peeled and cored

½ cup pear juice or nectar (found at health-food stores or in the ethnic food aisle)

2 teaspoons grated fresh ginger

1 teaspoon grated fresh lemongrass

Salt and ground black pepper to taste

1 small avocado, finely diced

1 plum tomato, finely diced

2 tablespoons crème fraîche

Juice of ½ lime

Place the mangoes and pears in a blender. Add the pear juice and puree until smooth. Add the ginger and lemongrass, and blend. Adjust seasoning with salt and pepper. If the soup is too thick, add a little water or a splash of white wine to thin it out.

Place the avocado and tomato in a small bowl and toss with salt and pepper. Mix the crème fraîche and lime juice in a separate bowl. Season with salt and pepper.

Ladle the soup into 6 chilled soup bowls. Place a dollop of the crème fraîche mixture in the center of each bowl and a spoonful of the avocado-tomato mixture on top. Serve immediately.

PER SERVING: 160 CALORIES • 1 G PROTEIN • 27 G CARBOHYDRATES • 6 G FAT

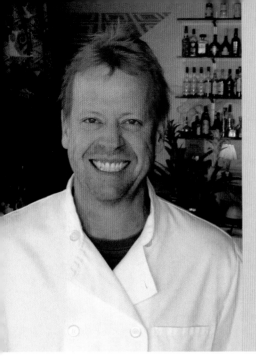

RICK MAHAN

Just a year after he started running, Rick Mahan ran his first 26.2. More impressive is that he finished the race, the San Francisco Marathon, in 3:51. Within 5 years the chef-owner of the Waterboy, a restaurant in Sacramento, California, completed his first 50-miler, the American River 50. "Immediately after the race, I felt thankful it wasn't the A.R. 51," says the chef, who also helms a pizzeria called One Speed, in honor of his other favorite pastime, cycling. Still, he's set his sights on the Western States 100, a 100-miler on trails in California's Sierra Nevada mountains. "Running is my alone time," says Mahan, who logs his weekly 40 miles solo but occasionally races with his colleagues. "The longer I run, the more time I have to myself." For more, go to waterboyrestaurant.com and onespeedpizza.com.

Potato Leek Soup with Steamed Clams

RECOVERY

This hearty soup is an example of the French and Italian influences at the Waterboy, Rick Mahan says. Leeks and other allium vegetables such as garlic and onion contain organosulfuric compounds that have been shown to protect against cancer. These vegetables also help stabilize blood sugar and blood pressure levels.

Makes 4 servings

PREP TIME: 15 MINUTES / COOK TIME: 15–20 MINUTES

2 tablespoons vegetable oil

2 cups sliced leeks

3 Yukon Gold potatoes, peeled and sliced (about 1½ pounds or 4 cups)

3 cloves garlic, minced

1 teaspoon chopped fresh thyme

1 teaspoon kosher salt

¼ teaspoon ground black pepper

3 cups water or chicken broth

⅓ cup cream, half-and-half, or whole milk (optional)

24 small fresh clams

2 slices bacon, diced

2 tablespoons sliced shallots

1 bunch watercress or arugula

Heat the oil in a heavy-bottomed saucepan. Add the leeks and cook for 4 minutes, stirring frequently. Add the potatoes, garlic, thyme, salt, and pepper and cook for 4 more minutes. Add 2½ cups of the water or broth and bring to a simmer. Cover and cook for 15 minutes or until the potatoes are breaking apart. Remove from the heat and crush the mixture gently with a whisk. Add the cream, if desired. Set aside. Steam the clams with the reserved ½ cup of water or chicken broth until the shells open, about 5 to 10 minutes. Add the steaming liquid (reserve the clams) to the soup. Brown the bacon in a separate pan. Add the shallots to the bacon and cook for 30 seconds. Add the watercress, stirring quickly to wilt. Ladle the soup into 4 bowls, divide the greens and bacon among the bowls, top with 6 clams each, and serve.

PER SERVING (BASED ON 4 SERVINGS, WITHOUT DAIRY):
350 CALORIES • 22 G PROTEIN • 43 G CARBOHYDRATES • 10 G FAT

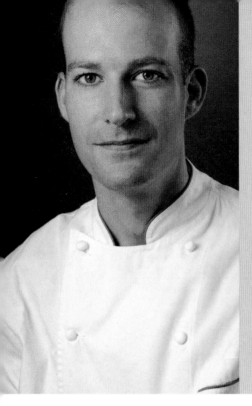

MATT CONNORS

When Matt Connors took a hiatus from working at a New York City restaurant to cook his way through Italy, it was an epiphany. "I realized I needed to be in the countryside to both run and cook better," he says. While searching for a spot to open a restaurant, Connors ran the Dublin, Rome, and New York City marathons, among others, and a month after opening his restaurant, the Lake House, in his hometown of Bay Shore, New York, he ran Boston. With 10 and counting 26.2s under his belt (and a PR of 3:05), Connors trains continually by running shorter distances every weekend, even if it's only a 5-K, and he cross-trains with karate. "It emphasizes intense stretching, ab and core training, and leg muscle strength exercises," Connors says. "I'd been reluctant to get into cross-training because I thought it would take away from my running ability, but it's had the opposite effect." For more, go to thelakehouserest.com.

Ribollita

TRAINING

"I lived in Italy for a year and fell in love with this traditional Tuscan bread soup," Matt Connors says. "I make this and keep it in the fridge for a week because it just gets better with time."

Italians make ribollita (which means "reboiled") from leftovers, and they cook the soup twice before eating it. It's loaded with carbs and protein, and the only fat comes from olive oil, which contains beneficial monounsaturated fats. Make the soup with whatever light-colored beans you have on hand. For more from Matt Connors, see pages 116, 132, and 136.

Makes 4 generous servings

PREP TIME: 20 MINUTES / COOK TIME: 1 HOUR 40 MINUTES

1 can (14 ounces) cannellini (or any white bean), drained and rinsed

¼ cup extra virgin olive oil

1 tablespoon chopped fresh garlic

1 tablespoon chopped fresh rosemary

1 large onion, chopped

2 ribs celery, chopped

1 carrot, chopped

1 bunch kale, roughly chopped

1 large Yukon Gold potato, diced

1 cup chopped canned tomatoes

2 cups chicken stock

3 slices day-old crusty white country bread

Salt and ground black pepper to taste

Reggiano Parmigiano cheese, grated (optional)

Mash 1 cup of the beans in a bowl with the back of a fork until smooth. Set aside. Heat ¼ cup oil in a heavy-bottomed pot for 1 minute. Add the garlic, rosemary, onion, celery, carrot, and kale and gently cook for 20 minutes, stirring occasionally. Add both the mashed and whole beans, potato, and tomatoes, and stock. Simmer gently for at least 1 hour. Add the bread and simmer until it's completely dissolved into the soup, about 10 minutes. Adjust seasoning with salt and pepper. Serve (preferably the next day), drizzled with olive oil and sprinkled with the grated cheese.

PER SERVING: 440 CALORIES • 6 G PROTEIN • 57 G CARBOHYDRATES • 17 G FAT

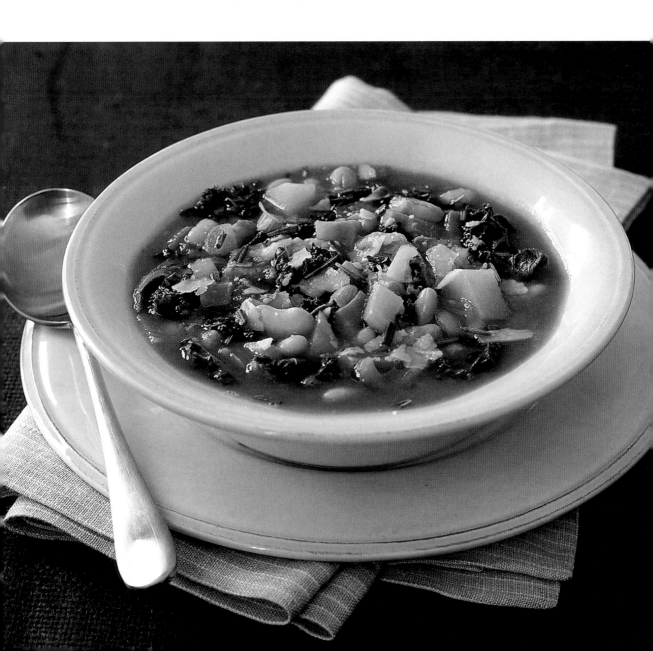

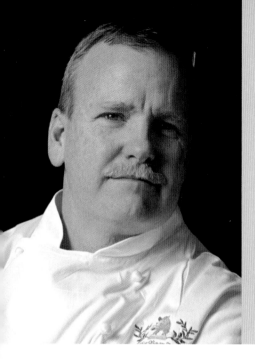

CHRISTOPHER SHEEHAN

It was Christopher Sheehan's daughter, Megan, who encouraged him to start running again, after he'd given it up for 15 years. In the process, Sheehan dropped 20 pounds and picked up a renewed appreciation for the flora and fauna near Blue Boar Inn, 20 minutes from Park City, Utah, where he had been working as the chef. While running the trails of the Wasatch Mountains with his border collie, he's spotted elk, moose, and a large coyote. "It followed me for half a mile," says the Los Angeles native. "Then I shouted and scared it off." Now the executive chef at Park Meadows Country Club in Heber City, Utah, he rides his mountain bike 10 miles round-trip to work, through Round Valley, and continues to hit running trails for 20 to 25 miles a week. For more, go to parkmeadowscc.com.

Shrimp and Artichoke Gazpacho   RECOVERY

A low-calorie, low-fat source of protein, shrimp are an excellent source for selenium, a cancer-fighting trace mineral, as well as vitamin D, which prevents bone loss and lowers the risk of heart disease and cancer, heart-healthy vitamin B$_{12}$, and omega-3 fatty acids. Artichokes are an excellent source of fiber; 1 medium artichoke provides 41 percent of your Daily Value and just 64 calories.

Makes 6 servings

PREP TIME: 15 MINUTES + 1 HOUR REFRIGERATION TIME

5 cups chopped tomatoes

1 clove garlic, minced

2 English cucumbers, peeled and diced

1 red bell pepper, roasted, peeled, seeded, and diced (or jarred)

¼ cup minced scallions

4 cups tomato juice

¼ cup bottled chili sauce

1 tablespoon prepared horseradish

¼ cup red wine vinegar

¼ cup fresh lemon juice

2 tablespoons Worcestershire sauce

2 tablespoons chopped fresh basil

2 tablespoons chopped fresh oregano

2 tablespoons chopped fresh parsley

2 cups diced precooked or grilled small bay shrimp

1 avocado, diced

1½ cups quartered artichoke hearts (drained)

Salt and black pepper to taste

Pinch of ground red pepper

In a large bowl, stir together all ingredients and refrigerate for at least 1 hour before serving.

PER SERVING: 260 CALORIES • 25 G PROTEIN • 30 G CARBOHYDRATES • 7 G FAT

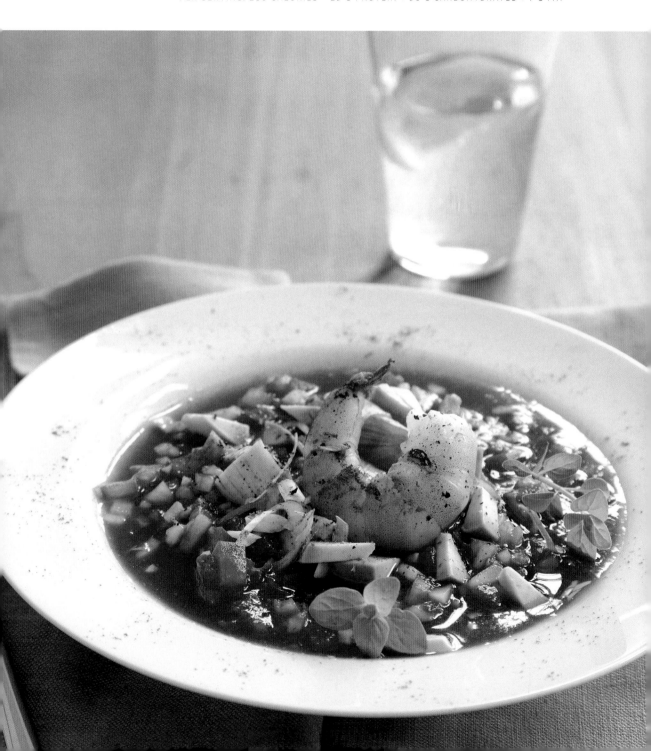

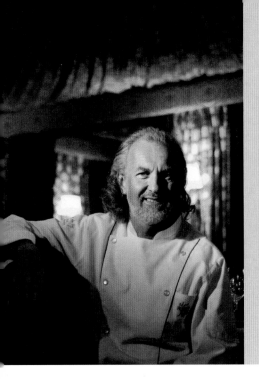

HUBERT KELLER

The challenge given to Hubert Keller was to devise vegan, fat-free recipes for inclusion in Dean Ornish, MD's book, *Eat More, Weigh Less*. As a Frenchman who grew up buttering cake molds in his father's patisserie, Keller's response was, "You're taking away everything that's French in me!" Still, the chef who oversees three restaurants in six locations, including Fleur de Lys in San Francisco, managed to develop low-fat cooking techniques for classic French dishes. He substitutes dried mushrooms sautéed in wine for bacon and favors pureed vegetables and garlic over cream and butter. Inspired, he decided to overhaul his own lifestyle. He began eating healthier and now counts a 6-mile loop from his Bay Area home as his favorite run. For more, go to fleurdelyssf.com.

Succulent Potato Stew with Asparagus and Shiitake Mushrooms

`RECOVERY`

Because of their starchiness and fiber content, the vegetables in this low-fat stew help provide a satisfying heartiness.

Makes 4 servings

PREP TIME: 25 MINUTES / COOK TIME: 60 MINUTES

6 new yellow potatoes (about 3 pounds), scrubbed and peeled

2 garlic cloves, finely minced

1 onion, coarsely minced

3 tablespoons coarsely minced carrot

3 tablespoons coarsely minced celery

1 small leek, finely julienned (use only the white bulb)

Salt and freshly ground pepper, to taste

1 cup dry white wine

2½ cups vegetable broth or water

1 sprig thyme

16 asparagus tips, 3½" long

½ tablespoon extra virgin olive oil

12 ounces shiitake mushroom caps, diced

2 tablespoons chives, finely minced

Slice the potatoes into ½" cubes, and empty them into a heavy saucepot. Season the garlic, onion, carrot, celery, and leek with salt and pepper, and add them to the pot. Add the wine, vegetable broth, and thyme, and mix gently. Add more water if any potatoes are not submerged. Bring the pot to a boil over medium-high heat. Cover and cook on low heat until the potatoes are fork-tender and the liquid is nearly cooked off, about 45 minutes.

While the potatoes cook, boil salted water in a saucepan and blanch the asparagus for 4 to 5 minutes, until tender. Transfer it immediately to an ice bath. When cool, drain and set aside. Just before the potato stew is cooked, heat the olive oil in a nonstick skillet. Add the mushrooms and sauté over medium heat for 4 to 5 minutes. Add the asparagus and sauté for about 2 more minutes. Season with salt and pepper. Garnish the stew with the asparagus and mushrooms. Sprinkle with the chives.

PER SERVING: 387 CALORIES • 12 G PROTEIN • 69 G CARBOHYDRATES • 2 G FAT

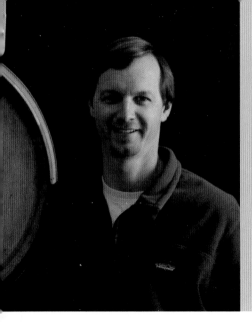

ANDREW MURRAY

Andrew Murray inherited a love of food and wine from his parents, who owned a restaurant and vineyard in California. To avoid inheriting another family trait—heart disease—he took up triathlons. "I love the endorphins and camaraderie," he says. "I compete because I get great pleasure from it." Murray began making his own Rhône-style wines after traveling to vineyards in France and Australia, and he swears by the invigorating 4- to 7-mile runs around his winery. "There is no better stress release than a nice run through the country," he says. For more, go to andrewmurrayvineyards.com.

Sweet Butternut Squash Soup

RECOVERY

"This is a great winter soup that provides tons of energy for muscles recovering from either a hard day at the winery or a hard day of training," Andrew Murray says. The creamy soup's slight natural sweetness pairs well with a crisp white wine, such as Murray's own Viognier or a New Zealand Sauvignon Blanc.

A 1-cup serving of butternut squash provides an average of 900 milligrams of potassium, critical for keeping hydrated and fueling recovery, and 6 grams of fiber, which helps fill you up and keeps you regular. The squash also is a good source of vitamin A (in the form of beta-carotene), which fights inflammation.

Makes 6 servings

PREP TIME: 15 MINUTES / COOK TIME: 1 HOUR 45 MINUTES

4 pounds butternut squash

Extra virgin olive oil for brushing squash +
   2 tablespoons

1 tablespoon unsalted butter

2 yellow onions, thinly sliced (about 4 cups)

3 cups low-sodium chicken stock

1 cup half-and-half

½ teaspoon chopped fresh thyme

½ teaspoon chopped fresh rosemary

½ teaspoon chopped fresh sage

1½ teaspoons chopped fresh flat-leaf
   parsley

Kosher salt and freshly ground black
   pepper

Preheat the oven to 400°F. Cut the squash in half and scoop out the seeds. Brush the flesh with oil and place cut-side down on a baking sheet. Roast for 1½ hours or until very soft. Let cool. Scoop the squash from the skin and set aside. Heat the butter with 2 tablespoons of olive oil in a pan over medium heat. Add the onions and cook until soft and golden, about 5 minutes. Puree the squash, onions, and 1 cup of the stock in a food processor, until smooth. Transfer the squash mixture to a large pot. Add the remaining chicken stock and heat the soup to a simmer, about 10 minutes. Add the half-and-half, thyme, rosemary, sage, and parsley. Season with salt and pepper and serve.

PER SERVING: 310 CALORIES • 8 G PROTEIN • 43 G CARBOHYDRATES • 15 G FAT

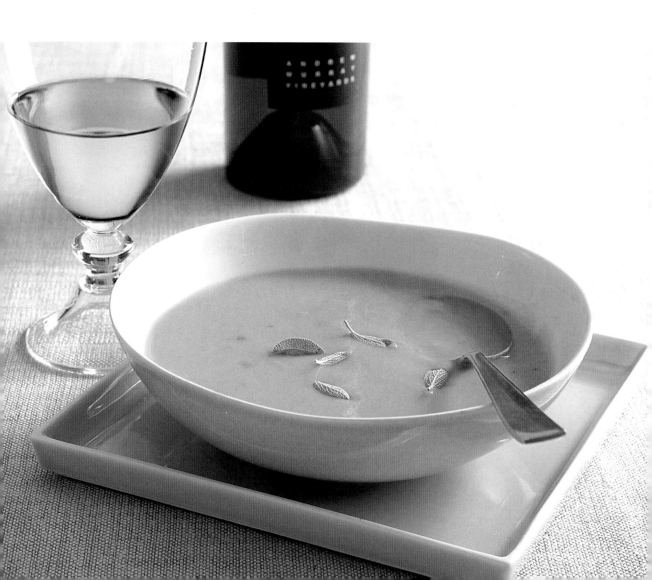

Arugula Salad

Andrew Dornenberg and Karen Page say the bitterness of arugula can be balanced with acidity, saltiness, and a touch of sweetness. Fresh leafy greens such as arugula, which is also known as rocket, are a great source of nutrients in a low-calorie package. Arugula provides vitamins A and C as well as folate, which helps lower levels of homocysteine, an amino acid in the blood that in excess has been linked to cardiovascular disease. Arugula also contains potassium, critical for balancing the body's fluids and for storing carbohydrates to use as fuel. For more from Andrew Dornenberg and Karen Page, see page 133.

Makes 4 servings

PREP TIME: 5 MINUTES

6 cups arugula

½ cup blue cheese, crumbled

1 pear, sliced

2 tablespoons extra virgin olive oil

Juice of ½ lemon

Salt and ground black pepper to taste

Mix the arugula with the cheese and pear, dress with the olive oil and lemon juice, and add salt and pepper to taste.

PER SERVING: 160 CALORIES • 5 G PROTEIN • 8 G CARBOHYDRATES • 12 G FAT

Baby Organic Field Greens with Blood Orange, Stilton Cheese, and Walnuts

Leafy greens are a good, low-calorie source of vitamins C and A as well as fiber. Blood oranges contain antioxidant anthocyanins that help reduce inflammation and protect against cancer, diabetes, and neurological diseases. They are also rich in vitamin C, folate, and fiber. Walnuts are a good source of heart-healthy omega-3 fatty acids. For more from Mark Monette, see pages 70 and 127.

Makes 2 servings

PREP TIME: 10 MINUTES

3 cups baby organic field greens, washed and dried

1 blood orange, segmented

2 tablespoons Stilton cheese, in pieces

¼ cup walnuts, toasted and coarsely chopped

3–4 tablespoons vinaigrette or extra virgin olive oil and balsamic vinegar to taste

Freshly ground black pepper

Toss the greens in a bowl with the blood orange segments, Stilton, and walnuts. Dress the salad with the vinaigrette and black pepper to taste, and serve immediately.

PER SERVING: 208 CALORIES • 6 G PROTEIN • 16 G CARBOHYDRATES • 15 G FAT

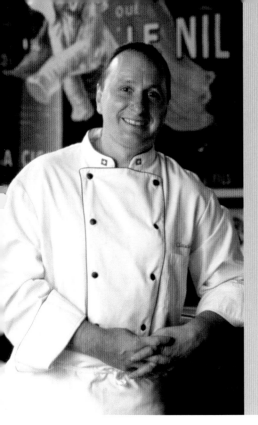

CLAUDE SOLLIARD

Like most runners on the night before the New York City Marathon, Claude Solliard loads up on pasta. But his noodles contain an unusual ingredient: seaweed. The executive chef at Seppi's in Manhattan uses a noodle made from a calcium-rich sea vegetable as the base for his unorthodox prerace dinner and for multiple dishes on his menu. "Kombu noodles don't contain flour, so they don't weigh me down, and their plain taste responds well to seasoning," says Solliard, who has run the five-borough marathon more than a dozen times. Postrace, the Swiss native indulges in a Turkish bath and massage, then works the dinner shift. While he's in the kitchen, he keeps his eye on the door, as marathon winners sometimes stop in. "We've served Martin Lel (2003), Hendrick Ramaala (2004), and Margaret Okayo (2001, 2003)," says Solliard. But you don't have to win to celebrate at Seppi's. Anybody who comes in on race day wearing a marathon medal will be poured a glass of Champagne on the house. For more, go to seppis.com.

Beef and Kombu Noodle Salad `TRAINING`

Common in Japanese dishes, low-calorie kombu seaweed is a good source for various vitamins and minerals, including calcium, vitamins A and B_1, magnesium, iron, potassium, and fiber.

Kombu noodles can be found under the Japanese Delight brand at Amazon.com, at McMahonsFarm. com, or at Asian groceries. You can also substitute cooked spaghetti for the kombu noodles. For more from Claude Solliard, see page 99.

Makes 6 servings

PREP TIME: 10 MINUTES / COOK TIME: 5 MINUTES

3 packets (6 ounces each) kombu noodles

2 tablespoons fresh lemon juice

3 teaspoons sesame oil

3 tablespoons soy sauce

2 cups cherry tomatoes, halved

2 cups avocado, diced (about 2 avocados)

1½ pounds flank or strip steak

Salt and white pepper to taste

2 endives

2 tablespoons chopped fresh basil

Open kombu noodles and rinse (no cooking required). Whisk together the lemon juice, sesame oil, and soy sauce in a large bowl. Add the kombu noodles, tomatoes, and avocados. Sauté the beef for about 5 minutes in a medium skillet over moderate heat, then add it to the noodle mixture. Season with the salt and white pepper to taste. Arrange the endive leaves on a wide plate to look like rays, leaving a circle in the middle. Place the noodle salad in the center, and top with basil.

PER SERVING: 300 CALORIES • 28 G PROTEIN • 10 G CARBOHYDRATES • 17 G FAT

Crab Salad with Avocado, Apple, and Green Beans

An excellent source of low-fat protein, crabmeat provides vitamins such as immune-boosting C and heart-healthy B_{12}. Like other seafoods, crabmeat contains omega-3 fatty acids, which boost cardiovascular health and brain function. You can also substitute lobster meat for the crab. Avocado contains monounsaturated fat that helps regulate blood cholesterol levels. Serve this salad on a bed of greens, or on a fresh roll for added carbs and calories. For more from Patricia Wells, see page 16, 104, 181, and 194.

Makes 4 servings

PREP TIME: 10 MINUTES / COOK TIME: 3–4 MINUTES

1½ cups green beans, trimmed at both ends, cut into ½" pieces

2 tablespoons coarse sea salt

1 cup 2% Greek-style yogurt

1 tablespoon Dijon mustard

¼ teaspoon fine sea salt

4 tablespoons minced fresh chives

1 Granny Smith apple, peeled and cubed

1 ripe avocado, peeled and cubed

8 ounces cooked lump crabmeat (about 1 cup)

Fill a large pot (fitted with a colander) with water. Bring to a rolling boil over high heat. Add the green beans and 2 tablespoons of salt, and cook until crisp-tender, 3 to 4 minutes. Remove the colander from the water. Rinse the beans with cold water so they cool quickly and stay green and crisp. Drain the beans and pat dry with a clean towel. Whisk together the yogurt, mustard, and salt in a large, shallow bowl. Add the green beans, chives, apple, avocado, and crabmeat. Toss carefully to evenly coat all the ingredients with the dressing, and serve.

PER SERVING: 220 CALORIES • 20 G PROTEIN • 17 G CARBOHYDRATES • 9 G FAT

JASON SERAYDARIAN

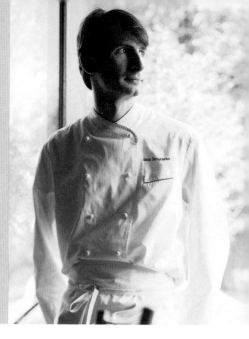

For Jason Seraydarian, cooking runs in the family. From 1900 to 1930, his great-grandfather ran Heermann's Bakery in Philadelphia, famous for its bread and ice cream. "My parents taught me to cook," he says. "It was lots of potted meals." Seraydarian followed in his family's footsteps by becoming a chef himself, and he helmed a Philadelphia restaurant before departing to New Jersey and launching a consulting business. Running is also a family affair for Seraydarian, who courted his wife during runs when they lived in New York City. The two-time New York City marathoner keeps fit by chasing after his two kids, cycling, and swimming. For more, go to jseraydarian.com.

Duck Breast and Beet Salad

`RECOVERY`

The duck in this dish provides protein for muscle recovery, while the fiber-rich beets contain potassium, which helps maintain fluid and electrolyte balance. You can use grilled chicken or grilled salmon instead of the duck. For more from Jason Seraydarian, see page 18.

Makes 2 servings

PREP TIME: 15 MINUTES / COOK TIME: 15 MINUTES

1 duck breast (6 to 8 ounces), fat trimmed

Salt and ground black pepper to taste

1 can (16 ounces) beets, drained

1 teaspoon chopped fresh tarragon

1 tablespoon chopped fresh mint

Grated peel and juice 1 orange

1 tablespoon red wine vinegar

1 teaspoon honey

1 teaspoon Dijon mustard

1 tablespoon extra virgin olive oil

2 cup baby greens

1 teaspoon aged balsamic vinegar

Clean the duck and cut small slits into the skin to allow the fat to drip out. Season liberally with salt and pepper, and sauté over high heat until medium-rare, about 5 to 7 minutes on each side, or until the skin is crispy and golden-brown. Allow the duck to cool, then slice.

In a large bowl, mix together the beets, tarragon, mint, orange peel, orange juice, vinegar, honey, mustard, and oil, and season with salt and pepper to taste. Place the greens in the center of the plate and drizzle with the balsamic vinegar. Spoon the beet salad on top of the greens, and arrange the duck around the salad.

PER SERVING: 290 CALORIES • 20 G PROTEIN • 27 G CARBOHYDRATES • 11 G FAT

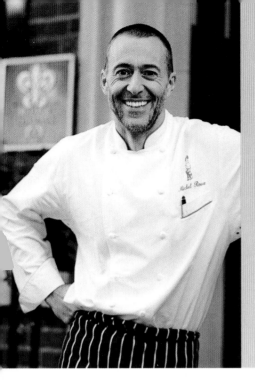

MICHEL ROUX JR.

Michel Roux Jr. can prepare an artichoke heart in less than 30 seconds. But he's more proud of his PR at the 2001 London Marathon, where he clocked 3:13. The executive chef of London's family-run Le Gavroche—which, in 1982, became the first U.K. restaurant to earn three Michelin stars—began racing in marathons more than a decade ago to offset the weight he'd gained after he quit smoking. With 17 marathons under his belt, Roux then went on to try an ultramarathon and finished the 2003 Le Périgord Noir, a 100-K race in Belvès, France, in 10:56. In search of healthy recipes to enjoy while training, Roux created enough of his own to fill a cookbook *The Marathon Chef.* "I wanted to prove that you can eat French food and keep fit at the same time," he says. For more, go to michelroux.co.uk.

Endive and Poached Egg Salad with Red Onions and Dry-Cured Bacon

RECOVERY

Michel Roux Jr. likes to refuel after a workout with a light salad such as this one. Eggs contain highly digestible protein, endive provides a good dose of the antioxidant beta-carotene, and walnuts are a good source of heart disease–preventing omega-3 fatty acids. Along with having antibacterial properties, red onions contain flavonoids and other compounds that have been shown to decrease inflammation, fight cancer and heart disease, and promote bone health.

Makes 6 servings

PREP TIME: 10 MINUTES / BAKE AND COOK TIME: 7–8 MINUTES

18 walnuts (about ½ cup)	6 eggs
1 tablespoon water	2–4 tablespoons white wine vinegar
4 tablespoons balsamic vinegar	12 very thin slices pancetta
6 tablespoons extra virgin olive oil	4 Belgian endives
Salt and ground black pepper to taste	2 red onions, thinly sliced

Preheat the oven to 400°F. Put the walnuts, water, vinegar, olive oil, salt, and pepper in a blender. Pulse to make the vinaigrette (makes about ½ cup).

Crack the eggs into separate cups, and gently pour them into unsalted boiling water with the 4 tablespoons of vinegar (about 2 tablespoons per quart of water). Cook for no more than 3 minutes for soft eggs. Remove them with a slotted spoon, and gently place them in ice water to halt the cooking. Drain, dry, and wrap each egg in 2 slices of pancetta.

Cut the endives at the base. Arrange the smaller leaves in a circle around each of 6 plates. Thinly slice the rest to put in the middle.

Intersperse the onion with the endive. Drizzle the walnut vinaigrette onto each plate. To reheat the eggs, place them in a lightly oiled dish and warm them in the preheated oven for 4 to 5 minutes. Place an egg in the center of each salad and serve.

PER SERVING: 308 CALORIES • 10 G PROTEIN • 8 G CARBOHYDRATES • 27 G FAT

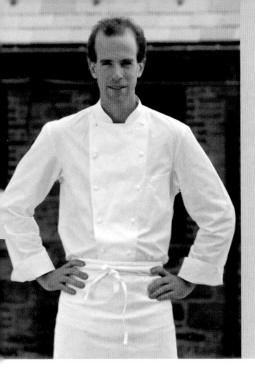

DAN BARBER

When Dan Barber works at his restaurant Blue Hill in New York City—where the Obamas dined during a quick trip—he runs along the busy West Side Highway. But his second restaurant, Blue Hill at Stone Barns in Pocantico Hills, New York, about 40 minutes north of the city, is on a former Rockefeller estate, and the New York City native can go for 30- to 40-minute runs on the property's quiet carriage trails. "It helps energize me for the evening rush," he says. For inspiration, this proponent of locally grown food (Stone Barns includes a greenhouse and working farm) listens to books on tape while he runs. One favorite: Aldo Leopold's 1949 classic of environmental conservation, *A Sand County Almanac.* "It's my running companion," he says. For more, go to bluehillfarm.com.

Kale Salad with Pine Nuts, Currants, and Parmesan

`RECOVERY`

Kale is an excellent source of potassium and vitamins A and C. Cruciferous vegetables like kale have been shown to fight cancer, particularly of the colon, breast, and bladder, thanks to phytochemicals called glucosinolates. The potent glucosinolate sulforaphane is released when cruciferous vegetables are chopped or chewed. If you can't find Tuscan kale, which has crinkly, pebbly leaves, use the smaller, tender leaves of regular kale.

Makes 6 servings

PREP TIME: 10 MINUTES + 1 HOUR 20 MINUTES MARINATING TIME

2 tablespoons dried currants

7 tablespoons white balsamic vinegar

1 tablespoon unseasoned rice vinegar

1 tablespoon honey

1 tablespoon extra virgin olive oil

1 teaspoon salt + additional for seasoning

2 bunches Tuscan kale (about 1 pound), center ribs and stems removed, leaves thinly sliced crosswise

2 tablespoons pine nuts, lightly toasted

Ground black pepper

Parmesan cheese shavings

Place the currants in a small bowl and add 5 tablespoons of the white balsamic vinegar. Soak for at least 1 hour, or overnight. Drain the currants.

Whisk the remaining 2 tablespoons of white balsamic vinegar, rice vinegar, honey, oil, and salt in a large bowl. Add the kale, currants, and pine nuts, then toss to coat. Let the mixture marinate for 20 minutes at room temperature, tossing occasionally. Season to taste with salt and pepper. Sprinkle the cheese shavings over the salad and serve.

PER SERVING: 110 CALORIES • 4 G PROTEIN • 14 G CARBOHYDRATES • 6 G FAT

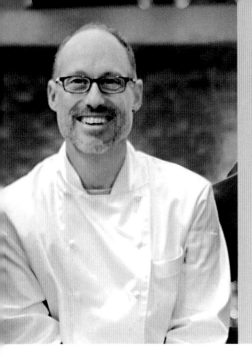

THOM FOX

The Acme Chophouse at AT&T Park, home of baseball's San Francisco Giants, isn't your typical steakhouse. That's because its executive chef, Thom Fox, isn't your typical meat-and-potatoes guy. He's a lifelong runner with a firm belief in the connection between food and health. "Running helped me see the clear link between how we eat, how we perform, and how we're connected to the earth," says Fox, whose 5-day-a-week exercise routine often includes 15-mile runs and 80-mile bike rides. But although Acme's menu focuses on local, organic produce and naturally raised fish and livestock, it doesn't mean you won't find fries. "Moderation in all things," says Fox. For more, go to acmechophouse.com.

Grilled Steak Salad

RECOVERY

Thom Fox says you can prepare this salad entirely on a grill or in an oven. Asparagus contains vitamin K, important for bone health and blood clotting, as well as folate and other B vitamins. One cup of asparagus contains about one-third of the Daily Value for vitamin C, an antioxidant. A member of the chicory family, which also includes endive and radicchio, escarole is a curly-leafed green with a milder taste than endive. Chicories are an excellent source of calcium, folate, vitamins A and C, iron, and potassium.

Makes 2 servings

PREP TIME: 10 MINUTES / COOK TIME: 15 MINUTES

8 ounces top sirloin steak

Salt and pepper to taste

1 tablespoon extra virgin olive oil

2 tablespoons white-wine vinegar

1 tablespoon water

2 teaspoons chopped fresh parsley

2 teaspoons chopped fresh oregano

1 teaspoon chili flakes

Coarse sea salt to taste

1 bunch asparagus, trimmed and blanched

1 small head escarole, halved, trimmed, and washed

(continued on page 58)

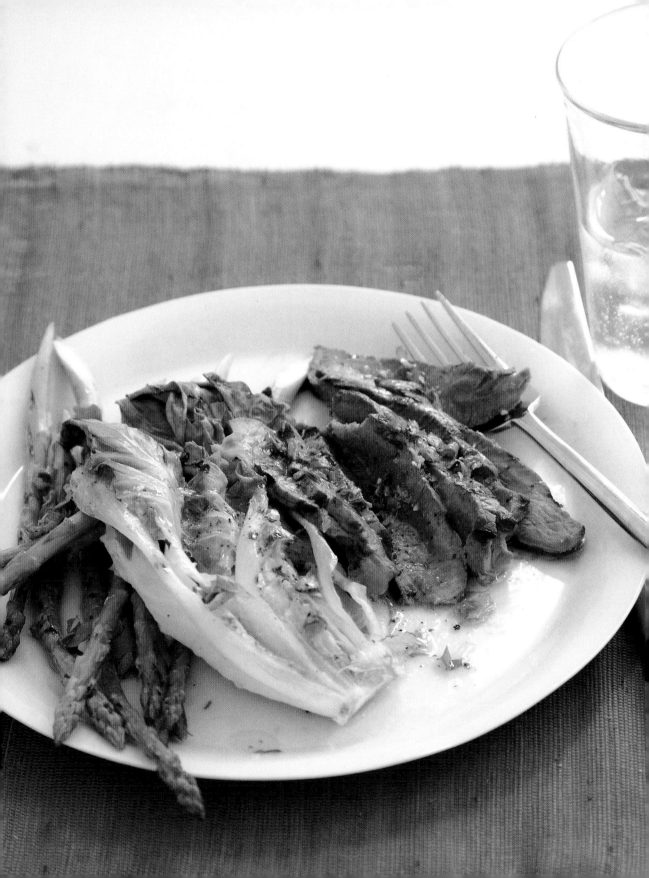

Season meat with salt and pepper. Grill until medium-rare at 140°F. Allow 12 to 15 minutes to cook, turning once. (Or roast in 400°F oven for 8 to 10 minutes.) Let rest for 5 minutes.

Make the chimichurri dressing by whisking together the olive oil, vinegar, water, parsley, oregano, and chili flakes. Add coarse sea salt to taste. Set aside.

Warm the blanched asparagus on the grill for a few minutes (or warm in a 300°F oven for a few minutes). Place escarole halves on the grill to wilt, about 3 minutes, turning once (or roast in a 400°F oven until wilted). Arrange escarole leaves on 2 plates and top with the asparagus and then the steak. Drizzle the dressing over the steak and asparagus and serve.

PER SERVING: 310 CALORIES • 33 G PROTEIN • 19 G CARBOHYDRATES • 13 G FAT

CLIFF PLEAU

Good thing Cliff Pleau has a head for numbers. On his daily 5-mile runs, the executive chef figures out dishes that clock in at 475 calories—or less—to serve at the Seasons 52 restaurant chain. The director of culinary development arrived at the magic number by dividing a typical daily intake of 2,200 to 2,400 calories by three, or 800 calories per meal. "The other 325 calories go to a starter and, at dinner, a glass of wine," he says. He eliminated creams and butters and emphasizes lean proteins, complex carbohydrates, and fruits and vegetables at their seasonal peak. Pleau practices what he preaches out of the kitchen, too. The Chicago native has run six marathons and is also an avid tae kwon do enthusiast and longtime wakeboarder. "The sparring in tae kwon do has strengthened the ligaments around my knees, which helps my running and wakeboarding," he says. "The sports complement one another." For more, go to seasons52.com.

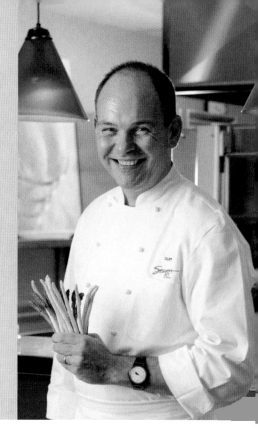

Roasted Corn Salad with Black Beans and Avocado

"When you roast corn in the husk, the silk comes off easily," Pleau says. Black beans are a great source of fiber and fat-free protein. Avocado contains heart-healthy unsaturated fats, as well as the antioxidants lutein, vitamin E, and vitamin C. Cumin seeds are a good source of iron and are important for energy production and immune function. In Indian cuisine, they also have been traditionally used to aid digestion. Toasting cumin seeds extracts their flavorful oils. To toast, place whole cumin seeds in a small, dry skillet and toast lightly over medium-high heat for 1 to 1½ minutes. Then grind the seeds to a fine powder in a coffee grinder or mince with a knife. For more recipes from Cliff Pleau, see pages 75 and 164.

Makes 8 cups

PREP TIME: 20 MINUTES + 5 MINUTES STAND TIME AND 4 HOURS MARINATING TIME / COOK TIME: 35 MINUTES (INCLUDES ROASTING CORN)

(continued on page 61)

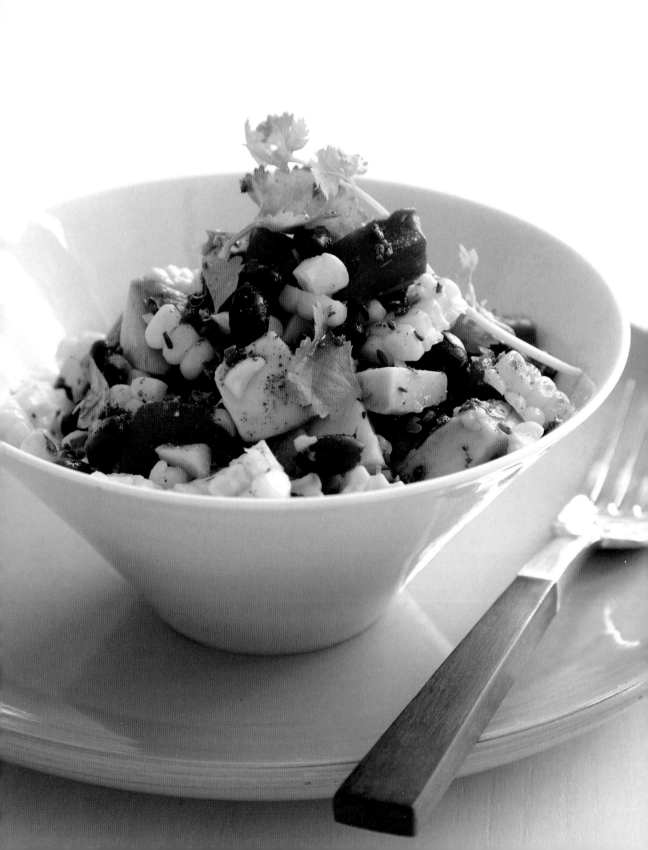

1 tablespoon extra virgin olive oil

1 tablespoon minced garlic

7 ears of corn, roasted (recipe below)

1 can (15 ounces) black beans, rinsed and
drained

1 red bell pepper, roasted, cut into ¼" dice
(can be store-bought, but fresh is best)

½ cup coarsely chopped cilantro

¼ cup lime juice

2 teaspoons blackening spice
or chili powder

2 teaspoons cumin, toasted and ground

2 teaspoons hot sauce, chipotle-style

1 teaspoon kosher salt

2 Hass avocados, peeled, pitted, and
cut in ½" chunks

Heat the oil in a sauté pan over medium-high heat. Add the garlic and cook, stirring frequently, until the garlic is golden-brown, 1 to 2 minutes.

Remove the garlic from the heat and place it in a medium bowl. Add the corn, beans, red pepper, cilantro, lime juice, blackening spice, cumin, hot sauce, and salt. Stir together until well combined. Gently fold in the chunks of avocado.

Let the salad marinate for 4 hours before serving.

PER SERVING: 216 CALORIES • 7 G PROTEIN • 32 G CARBOHYDRATES • 9 G FAT

Roasted Corn

Makes about 6 cups

7 ears yellow corn, in husk

Wash the corn in husks in cold water, then place on a baking sheet.

Roast for 30 minutes at 425°F. Cool to room temperature for 30 minutes. Peel off the husks and all silk strands.

Stand the corn on end and use a sharp knife to slice off the corn kernels.

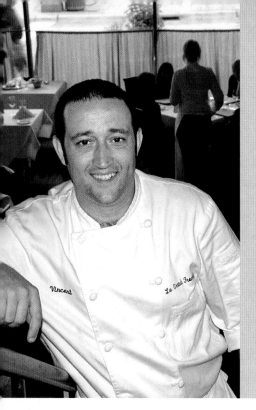

VINCENT FRANCOUAL

Vincent Francoual grew up bicycling the hills in a small town in southwestern France. As a teen, he started running while enlisted in the French Army. So as an adult, after he moved to Minneapolis and his doctor suggested he try swimming to help ease back pain, Francoual realized he now had the skills to tackle a new sport: triathlons. "For my first triathlon in 2004, I wanted pressure to make sure I would train and finish," says Francoual. He registered for the Life Time Fitness Triathlon in Minneapolis and organized a team of chefs to raise funds for Fraser, a local nonprofit that helps children with special needs. Each year since then, Francoual has raced the Olympic-distance triathlon and raised money for Fraser. In 2009, he broke 2 records: He earned a 2:47 PR for the 1.5-K swim, 40-K bike ride, and 10-K run, and his PR for fund-raising $51,000. For more, go to vincentarestaurant.com.

Salad Niçoise

`RECOVERY`

Vincent Francoual says this traditional salad is the perfect light meal after a warm-weather training session. "It's refreshing and healthy with the right balance of vegetables, starch, and protein," he says. "It's very easy to make and digest." For more from Vincent Francoual, see pages 90 and 188.

Makes 4 servings

PREP TIME: 15 MINUTES

1 head Bibb or romaine lettuce

2 ripe tomatoes, cut into 6 wedges

4 cooked Red Bliss potatoes, quartered

½ cup green beans, blanched

4 hard-boiled eggs, quartered

4 teaspoons pitted and chopped cured
   black olives

½ cup canned tuna in water

8 anchovy fillets

2 teaspoons Dijon mustard

3 teaspoons red-wine vinegar

Salt

1 cup extra virgin olive oil

To make the salad, arrange the lettuce leaves on the bottom of a bowl. Place the tomatoes, potatoes, green beans, eggs, and olives all around. Place the tuna in the center of a bowl and top it with the anchovies. To make the vinaigrette, mix together the mustard, vinegar, and salt; slowly whisk in the oil. Drizzle 4 tablespoons of the vinaigrette over the salad, and serve.

PER SERVING: 330 CALORIES • 18 G PROTEIN • 13 G CARBOHYDRATES • 23 G FAT

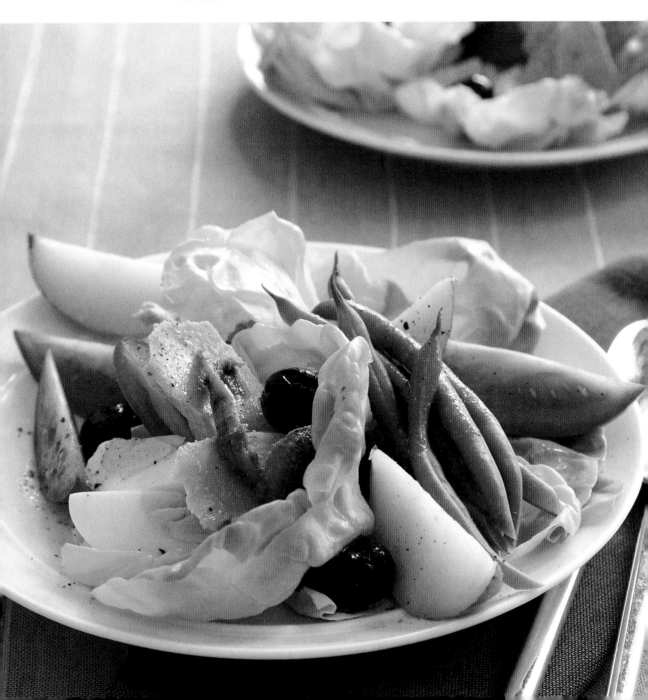

Salad of Port-Poached Figs with Point Reyes Blue Cheese

Dried figs are an excellent source of fiber and other nutrients. One serving of six figs contains 5 grams of fiber or 20 percent of the Daily Value, as well as 6 percent of the Daily Value each for calcium and iron. For more from James Boyce, see page 34.

Makes 4 servings

PREP TIME: 20 MINUTES / COOK TIME: 20–30 MINUTES

16 whole mission figs, dried

1 cup port

2 tablespoons balsamic vinegar

2 tablespoons orange juice

2 tablespoons brown sugar

1 stick cinnamon

1 whole star anise

1 Gala apple

2 cups assorted baby greens

1 teaspoon chopped chives

1 tablespoon extra virgin olive oil

Salt and pepper to taste

$\frac{1}{2}$ cup crumbled Point Reyes (or other creamy-style) blue cheese

Trim the stems of the figs and cut in half lengthwise. In a medium saucepan, combine the figs, port, vinegar, orange juice, brown sugar, cinnamon, and star anise. Bring to a simmer and cook for 20 to 30 minutes, or until the liquid reduces by two-thirds (makes about $\frac{1}{3}$ cup).

Thinly slice the apple and place in a medium mixing bowl. Add the greens and chives. Season with olive oil, salt, and pepper. Mix well.

Place equal amounts of salad in the middle of 4 salad plates. Remove the fig halves from the cooking liquid and place around each salad. Drizzle the liquid from cooking the figs around each plate and over the salad. Top with crumbled cheese and serve with crusty bread.

PER SERVING: 343 CALORIES • 6 G PROTEIN • 48 G CARBOHYDRATES • 9 G FAT

Shaved Brussels Sprout Salad

"Brussels sprouts earned their bad name mainly from the mushy, overcooked, underseasoned versions we were forced to eat when we were young," Hugh Acheson says. He created this simple salad as a fresh take on the much-maligned vegetable.

Brussels sprouts are an excellent source of vitamin K, critical for blood clotting and bone health. Like other cruciferous vegetables such as broccoli and cabbage, they contain the cancer-fighting phytochemical sulforaphane. They are also a good source of fiber. For another recipe from Hugh Acheson, see page 68.

Makes 10 servings (1 cup each)

PREP TIME: 25 MINUTES

2 teaspoons Dijon mustard

5 tablespoons extra virgin olive oil

2 tablespoons walnut oil

2 tablespoons lemon juice

2 teaspoons sherry vinegar

1 tablespoon finely chopped parsley

Salt and ground black pepper to taste

2 pounds Brussels sprouts, shaved thinly by hand or on a small mandoline

1 cup roasted peanuts, slightly broken up

1 cup shaved Pecorino Romano cheese (or Parmesan)

½ cup chopped flat leaf parsley

Whisk the Dijon mustard in a bowl and slowly add the olive and walnut oils to emulsify. If it gets too thick, dilute it with a touch of water toward the end.

When the oils are all incorporated, add the lemon juice and vinegar and then finish with the parsley, salt, and pepper.

Shave the Brussels sprouts into thin slices using a sharp knife or a small mandoline.

Place the shaved Brussels sprouts, peanuts, cheese, and parsley in a salad bowl and lightly dress with mustard vinaigrette to taste. Toss and serve.

PER SERVING: 257 CALORIES • 9 G PROTEIN • 12 G CARBOHYDRATES • 20 G FAT

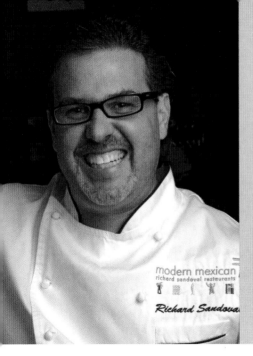

RICHARD SANDOVAL

As a young adult, Richard Sandoval had hopes of becoming a professional tennis star. But after a tough stint on the European circuit, the Mexico City native says he turned to what he really enjoys—cooking. Sandoval is the chef-owner of 15 Latin- and Asian-style restaurants in the United States, Mexico, and Dubai. Juggling restaurants in three countries has forced Sandoval to fine-tune his exercise routine. "Tennis is hard to manage with my travel schedule," he says, "so I started running. Wherever I go, I know where the closest gym is." Most mornings he can squeeze in 3 to 5 miles, usually while listening to Latin music, especially fast-tempo mariachi. For more, go to modernmexican.com.

Shrimp Noodle Salad

`TRAINING`

This Asian-Latin dish contains ginger, which reduces inflammation and fights cancer, as well as jalapeño chiles, which are rich in vitamins C and A. Instead of shrimp, you can use grilled beef, chicken, or tofu. For more from Richard Sandoval, see pages 126 and 169.

Makes 2 servings

PREP TIME: 30 MINUTES / COOK TIME: 5 MINUTES

3 ounces bean-thread vermicelli noodles

6 medium shrimp, peeled, cooked, and cooled

1 clove garlic, finely chopped

3 tablespoons chopped roasted peanuts

¼ tablespoon freshly squeezed lemon juice

1 tablespoon rice wine vinegar

½ tablespoon sesame oil

⅛ cup canola oil

¼ tablespoon fish sauce

½ tablespoon honey

¼ cup peeled and julienned green papaya

¼ cup peeled and julienned mango

1 tablespoon finely chopped basil

1 tablespoon finely chopped mint

1 tablespoon finely chopped cilantro

¾ tablespoon finely chopped fresh ginger

1 tablespoon thinly sliced scallions (green part only)

1 tablespoon thinly sliced jalapeño chili pepper

2 tablespoons thinly sliced shallots

Cilantro leaves and black sesame seeds to garnish

Place 2 cups of water in a medium saucepan and bring to a boil. Add the noodles and cook for 3 minutes. Strain and cool the noodles with cold water. Drain again, and set aside. Slice the shrimp lengthwise and add to the noodles, along with the garlic and peanuts. Add the papaya, mango, basil, mint, cilantro, ginger, scallions, jalapeño pepper, shallots, and the sesame vinaigrette. (To make the vinaigrette, whisk together $\frac{1}{4}$ tablespoon lemon juice, 1 tablespoon rice wine vinegar, $\frac{1}{2}$ tablespoon sesame oil, and $\frac{1}{8}$ cup canola oil. Mix in $\frac{1}{4}$ tablespoon fish sauce and $\frac{1}{2}$ tablespoon honey). Garnish salad with cilantro leaves and black sesame seeds.

PER SERVING: 470 CALORIES • 8 G PROTEIN • 55 G CARBOHYDRATES • 25 G FAT

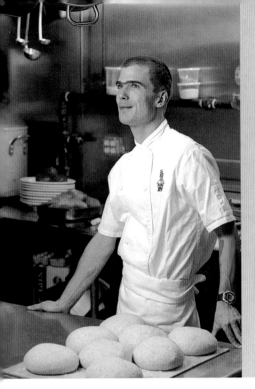

HUGH ACHESON

Hugh Acheson studied political philosophy in college. "I liked it because it was esoteric, and reading Kierkegaard seemed cool," he says. Then a simple truth dawned on him: "No one makes any money doing that." So instead Acheson turned his part-time dishwashing job into an award-winning career. He credits chef-mentors for teaching him cooking techniques in Ottawa, his hometown, and in San Francisco. Now Acheson is the chef at his own restaurant, Five & Ten, in Athens, Georgia, a place so personal and laid-back it's not unusual for the chef to answer the phone himself. Although Acheson says he's kept on his toes at the restaurant, he manages to squeeze in brief runs and games of tennis. He also recently opened a second Athens restaurant, the National, where his friend Peter Dale, another runner, is the chef. For more, go to fiveandten.com and thenationalrestaurant.com.

Tomato Salad

`QUICK AND EASY` `TRAINING`

The tomatoes in this simply prepared salad provide a good dose of vitamins C and A. The arugula adds iron, a crucial mineral athletes need to keep energy levels high. For more from Hugh Acheson, see page 65.

Makes 4 servings

PREP TIME: 20 MINUTES

2 pounds ripe, heirloom tomatoes, cored
    and thinly sliced into rounds (can
    substitute plum tomatoes)

Salt to taste

¼ pound (about 4 cups) arugula

2 tablespoons extra virgin olive oil

1 tablespoon balsamic vinegar

1 teaspoon fresh lemon juice

8 large, fresh basil leaves

¼ pound chunk of Parmigiano Reggiano

Freshly ground pepper

Place the tomatoes in a single layer on a cookie sheet. Season them lightly with the salt and set the sheet aside (do not refrigerate).

Toss the arugula with 1 tablespoon of the olive oil, the balsamic vinegar, and the lemon juice, and season very lightly with salt. Toss.

Layer the salad in this order: tomato, arugula, basil, tomato. You should have 3 levels of tomato and 2 levels of everything else. Use a peeler to shave pieces of cheese over the top to taste, drizzle with the remaining oil, and finish with freshly ground pepper.

PER SERVING: 226 CALORIES • 13 G PROTEIN • 12 G CARBOHYDRATES • 15 G FAT

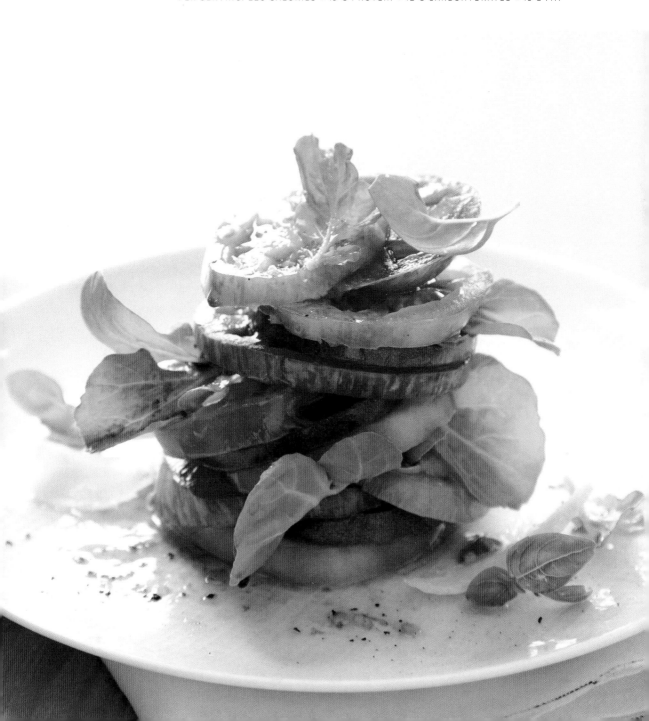

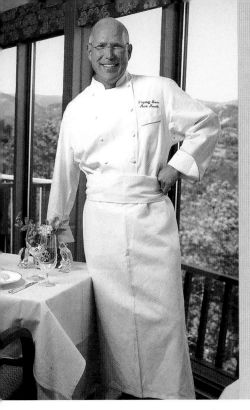

MARK MONETTE

Mark Monette always knew he wanted to work in a restaurant, but 30 years ago, being a chef wasn't glamorous. "It was considered a dirty job," says the runner and cyclist who now cooks 6,000 feet above Boulder, Colorado, in his family's restaurant, Flagstaff House. The chef and his brother also oversee the restaurant Monettes, featuring American French food, in the Mauna Kea Beach Hotel on the Big Island of Hawaii. "When I'm in Hawaii, I run to work on the coast in exactly 54 minutes, on a route that is part trail, part back road," says Monette, who logs 45 to 65 miles weekly. "It's a great way to start the day—in 80-degree weather watching whales jump in the water." Still, the marathoner, who finished the 2008 New York City Marathon in 3:34 a year after having foot surgery, prefers Colorado for optimal training. "The hills and altitude make it happen," he says. For more, go to flagstaffhouse.com.

Warm Salad of Alaskan Halibut and Arugula

`RECOVERY`

For a postworkout summer meal, Mark Monette likes a warm salad. "The halibut is lean and low in calories," he says. The garlic in it helps lower cholesterol, and the arugula and green peppers contain cancer-fighting beta carotene and vitamin C to boost immunity. For more from Mark Monette, see pages 47 and 127.

Makes 4 servings

PREP TIME: 55 MINUTES / COOK TIME: 30 MINUTES

4 teaspoons balsamic vinegar, reduced

4 halibut fillets, 6 to 8 ounces each

½ teaspoon salt

½ teaspoon white pepper

1 tablespoon salad oil

6 ounces arugula (about 4 packed cups)

1 roasted red or yellow sweet pepper, diced

1 heirloom tomato, cut into wedges

6 baby artichokes, cooked and quartered

3 tablespoons chopped Niçoise olives

3 cloves roasted garlic per salad

2 tablespoons extra virgin olive oil

1 teaspoon white truffle oil (optional)

6–8 croutons per salad

(continued on page 72)

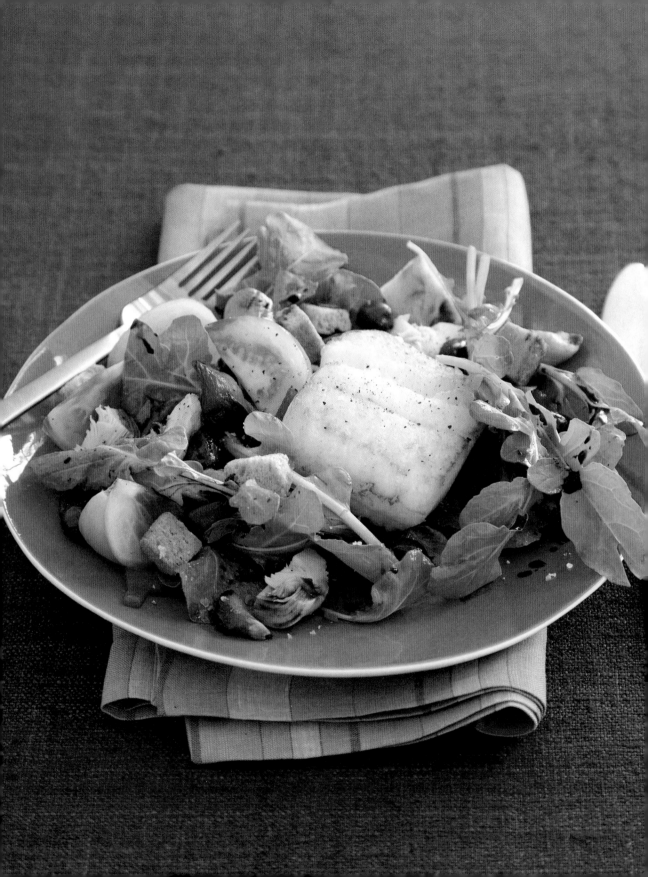

Balsamic reduction:

Add ½ quart of balsamic vinegar to a saucepan over a low flame in a slow simmer, allowing it to reduce until it has a syrupy consistency, about 20 minutes. Remove and chill. The syrup will get a little thicker as it chills. (Store in a squirt bottle in the refrigerator. It will keep for 1 month.)

Halibut:

Coat a grill rack with cooking spray and preheat the grill. Season the halibut with salt and white pepper, and brush it with salad or cooking oil (about 1 capful). Grill or sauté over medium flame until the flesh is all white (not gray) and flaky, about 6 minutes per side if fish is ¾" thick.

Salad:

While the halibut is cooking, mix the arugula, pepper, tomato, artichokes, olives, and garlic, dress with olive oil (and optional truffle oil), and toss. Arrange on 4 plates, drizzle each with 1 teaspoon of balsamic syrup. Add the croutons. Place a halibut fillet on top of each salad.

PER SERVING: 360 CALORIES • 39 G PROTEIN • 18 G CARBOHYDRATES • 13 G FAT

Baked Ricotta with Creamy Pesto Sauce

Part-skim ricotta is an excellent source of calcium and protein. It also contains vitamin A, iron, phosphorous, and selenium, a trace mineral that has been shown to fight cancer. For more from Giancarla Bodoni, see page 85.

Makes 16 appetizers or 8 side-dish servings

PREP TIME: 20 MINUTES / COOK AND BAKE TIME: 45 MINUTES

Baked Ricotta

2 pounds whole-milk ricotta

1½ cups whole milk

3 eggs

¼ teaspoon nutmeg

Salt and pepper

¾ cup pine nuts, finely chopped

Preheat oven to 325°F.

Place the ricotta in a mixer. Mix at medium speed while adding the milk. Add the eggs, one at a time. Season with nutmeg and salt and pepper to taste. Mix until the ingredients are well incorporated and the mixture is creamy.

Cut a piece of parchment paper to fit a 9″ spring-form pan. Grease the pan and the paper with butter. Fill the pan with the ricotta mixture. Cover with the chopped pine nuts and bake until golden, approximately 30 to 40 minutes, or until a knife inserted comes out clean.

Serve at room temperature with creamy pesto sauce (see below).

Pour the creamy pesto onto a plate. Slice the ricotta into 16 pieces and place the slices on top of the pesto. Drizzle with olive oil and serve warm.

Creamy Pesto Sauce

½ cup pine nuts

1 small garlic clove

1 cup extra virgin olive oil

Salt and pepper to taste

1½ cups fresh basil leaves

¾ cup half-and-half

Place the pine nuts, garlic, olive oil, and salt and pepper in a blender and process. Begin to add the basil leaves and process quickly until smooth. Do not overprocess or the basil will become dark.

Combine the half-and-half and pesto. Reduce to medium heat and cook until it is thickened. Add salt and pepper to taste.

PER SERVING: 308 CALORIES • 10 G PROTEIN • 5 G CARBOHYDRATES • 28 G FAT

Cauliflower Flan

Maria Hines says this vegetable flan is a nice accimpaniment to grilled meat or seafood. Besides being a great source of vitamin C—1 cup of boiled cauliflower contains close to 100 percent of the Daily Value for the antioxidant—cauliflower is a good source of the phytonutrient sulforaphane, which has been shown to fight cancer. For more from Maria Hines, see page 137.

Makes 4 servings

PREP TIME: 20 MINUTES / COOK TIME: 1 HOUR 10 MINUTES

1 head cauliflower, cut into florets

2 whole branches fresh parsley

2 branches fresh thyme

1 bay leaf

1½ cups whole milk

Salt and ground white pepper, to taste

2 large eggs, beaten

1 tablespoon butter, softened

Blanch the cauliflower in boiling water for several minutes until tender. Drain. Puree in a blender or food processor until smooth. Make a bouquet garni by placing the parsley, thyme, and bay leaf into a small square cheesecloth and securing the pouch with a piece of clean string or twine.

Add the cauliflower puree to a medium saucepan with the milk and bouquet garni. Let it steep over medium-low heat for 30 minutes. Season with the salt and pepper to taste. Discard the bouquet garni and strain the mixture through a fine-meshed sieve into a large bowl.

Beat the eggs in a separate large bowl. Slowly add about ¼ cup of the cauliflower mixture while whisking to temper the eggs and prevent them from curdling. Set aside.

Butter 4 (6-ounce) ramekins and set them in a shallow baking pan. Pour the custard into the 4 ramekins. Cover the ramekins with a sheet of parchment paper (1 sheet to cover all 4 is fine). Place the baking dish with the ramekins in the oven. Pour hot water into the baking dish to surround the outside of the ramekins so that the water is about halfway up the sides of the ramekins. This creates a water bath and helps the custard cook more gently.

Bake for 25 to 30 minutes or until the flans are set. Remove them from the oven.

To serve, gently slide the blade of a paring knife along the edge of the ramekin to loosen the flan, and tip over onto a dinner plate.

PER SERVING: 150 CALORIES • 9 G PROTEIN • 12 G CARBOHYDRATES • 8 G FAT

Grilled Spring Asparagus with Oven-Roasted Tomato Salsa

One cup of asparagus contains about a third of the Daily Value for vitamin C, a potent antioxidant. It is also an excellent source of bone-building vitamin K, heart-healthy folate, and vitamins A and B. For more from Cliff Pleau, see pages 59 and 164.

Makes 4 servings

PREP TIME: 15 MINUTES / BAKE AND COOK TIME: 20 MINUTES

1 pound trimmed fresh asparagus

Pepper to taste

2 tablespoons extra virgin olive oil

6 plum tomatoes

4 tablespoons red wine vinegar

1½ teaspoons crushed garlic

Salt and black pepper to taste

3 tablespoons chopped, fresh basil

4 ounces feta cheese + 2 ounces for garnish, crumbled

3 ounces (⅓ cup) kalamata olives, pitted and chopped

2 cups large-cut croutons

1 lemon, peeled and juiced

Blanch asparagus in boiling, salted water for 30 seconds and plunge into cold water to halt the cooking process. Season with pepper and 1 tablespoon of the olive oil.

Cut the tomatoes in half lengthwise. Toss in a bowl with the remaining tablespoon of olive oil, 2 tablespoons of the vinegar, 1 teaspoon of the crushed garlic, and pepper to taste. Toss together with half the basil. Roast on a baking sheet at 400°F for 15 minutes. Let cool.

Cut the oven-roasted tomatoes into chunks. Place them in a bowl and add the 4 ounces of feta, olives, lemon peel, the remaining ½ teaspoon garlic, and the remaining basil, and season it with salt and pepper.

Roast the asparagus in a 400°F oven for 3 to 4 minutes. Remove and drizzle with the lemon juice. Arrange the asparagus on 4 plates. Toss the croutons into the salsa and spoon over the asparagus. Top with the remaining 2 ounces of feta and the remaining 2 tablespoons of vinegar.

PER SERVING: 330 CALORIES • 11 G PROTEIN • 22 G CARBOHYDRATES • 23 G FAT

Guacamole

"Traditionally there's no lime juice in guacamole, but I found the citrus adds zest," Ivy Stark says. Serve the guacamole with warm tortillas. Avocado is an excellent source of the healthy, monounsaturated fat known as oleic acid (also found in olive oil). This kind of fat boosts levels of high-density lipoprotein (HDL or so-called "good" cholesterol) while reducing levels of low-density lipoprotein (LDL known as "bad" cholesterol). Avocados also provide the antioxidants lutein, vitamin E, and vitamin C.

Jalapeños contain vitamins C and A as well as capsaicin, the compound that gives chile peppers their heat and that may help fight cancer. For more from Ivy Stark, see pages 6 and 114.

Makes 4 cups

PREP TIME: 20 MINUTES

5 ripe Hass avocados, quartered, seeded, and peeled

6 tablespoons chopped cilantro

1 medium red onion, diced

2–4 (or to taste) jalapeño chile peppers, stemmed, seeded, and finely diced

3 tablespoons freshly squeezed lime juice

1 teaspoon salt

½ teaspoon freshly ground black pepper

3–4 fresh lettuce leaves

1–2 tomatoes, sliced

Place the avocado quarters in a mixing bowl. Mash with a potato masher or fork until chunky. Add the cilantro, onion, jalapeños, lime juice, salt, and pepper, and combine with a fork. Mound on a bed of lettuce and garnish with sliced tomatoes and cracked black pepper. Serve with warm corn tortillas.

PER SERVING: 200 CALORIES • 3 G PROTEIN • 12 G CARBOHYDRATES • 18 G FAT

PAUL MULLER

When the restaurant chain P.F. Chang's began sponsoring Arizona's Rock 'n' Roll Marathon, its top chef at the time, Paul Muller, didn't get it: What's Chinese food got to do with running? Then the Long Island native started running, completing two Rock 'n' Roll Half-Marathons. "High-carbohydrate, high-protein dishes are what make Chinese food," he says. "It's perfect for runners." Muller introduced low-fat, low-sodium interpretations of such Chinese-restaurant staples as Kung Pao Chicken to P.F. Chang's Training Table Menu, which was vetted by Olympian and avid cook Deena Kastor.

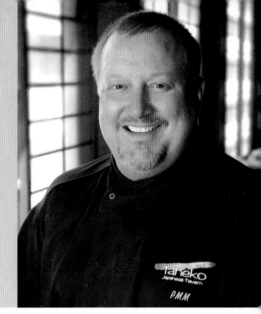

Sizzle Fish

RECOVERY

The "sizzle" (or light "poaching") comes from hot canola oil spooned over the sushi-grade fish, and the seasoning—ponzu (citrus) sauce, chives, garlic—gives the dish a light but tangy flavor. Find ponzu sauce at Asian groceries or gourmet markets. For more from Paul Muller, see page 102.

Makes 2 servings

PREP TIME: 20 MINUTES / COOK TIME: 5 MINUTES

6 ounces sushi grade halibut or salmon, slightly frozen

½ teaspoon minced ginger

⅛ teaspoon minced garlic

¼ teaspoon sliced chives

¼ teaspoon grated lemon peel

¼ teaspoon black sesame seeds

¼ teaspoon white sesame seeds

Okinawa salt to taste (or sea salt or fine-grain kosher salt to taste)

2 tablespoons blended sesame oil (or extra virgin olive oil)

2 tablespoons ponzu sauce

4 tablespoons micro greens

Place a plate in the refrigerator to chill. Cut the fish into ⅛" slices (about 7 slices). Slightly frozen fish cuts easier; use a very sharp knife. Arrange the slices in a circular pattern on the chilled plate. Sprinkle the ginger, garlic, chives, lemon peel, black and white sesame seeds, and salt over the fish slices. In separate small skillets, heat the sesame oil and ponzu sauce until hot. When the oil is smoking, spoon it over the fish slices—you should hear a loud sizzle. Spoon the ponzu over the fish. Place the micro greens in the middle of the plate.

PER SERVING (USING HALIBUT): 220 CALORIES • 18 G PROTEIN • 0 G CARBOHYDRATES • 16 G FAT

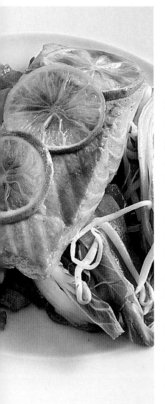

Mains

Carbohydrates, fat, and protein: These three nutrients are essential to every athlete's diet. To fuel muscles, your body requires carbs and fat. Carbs help shore up supplies of glycogen, the biggest energy source for your muscles. But for long workouts, you also need protein, since carbohydrate stores will begin to be depleted after about an hour. Protein also helps repair muscle damage and helps the body recover from exercise.

Ideally, athletes should consume a mix of carbs and protein within 30 to 60 minutes after a strenuous workout. A ratio of 4 grams of carbs to 1 gram of protein is a good rule of thumb. But remember that not all proteins, carbs, and fats are created equal: Aim for low-fat protein (think skinless chicken, lean meats, eggs, fish, soy); high-quality carbs (such as whole grains, beans, fruit, vegetables); and heart-healthy fats (like the mono- and polyunsaturated fats found in olive oil, nuts, and avocado).

That's where the recipes in this section come in. Food Network star Bobby Flay's Marathon Fettuccine is the perfect pre-race meal, with pan sautéed shrimp atop charred tomatoes and fettuccine. *Hell's Kitchen* star Gordon Ramsay's Pancetta Spaghetti is a simple, five-ingredient dish flavored with cured pork belly, garlic, and olive oil.

Cookbook author Devin Alexander's Superstuffed Steak Soft Taco is satisfying yet surprisingly lean, while salmon is a favorite protein for many of the chefs, who present it baked, grilled, and on top of pasta. Flavorful, easy to cook, and filled with omega-3 fatty acids, the fish is the athlete's no-brainer protein.

Vegetarians will appreciate many of the pasta options and two unconventional sandwiches: New York City chef Simpson Wong replaced bread with eggplant for his Eggplant Sandwich; and Boston pastry chef Tuesday Evans created a panini combining brie, chocolate, and olives. The unexpectedly tasty combination of sweet, briny, and savory surprised even our recipe testers.

Baked Macaroni and Artisanal Cheese
with Chorizo and Piquillo Peppers

Brown Rice with Blood Oranges and Raisins

Bucatini with Merguez Sausage

Fettuccine Paolo

Linguine with Genovese Pesto

Marathon Fettuccine in Charred
Tomato Sauce and Shrimp

Vincent's Mushroom Risotto

Orecchiette Carbonara with Chicken and
Broccoli

Pancetta Spaghetti

Pasta Mediterranée

Penne Arrabbiata

Rigatoni with Early Asparagus
and Shiitake Mushrooms

Rotelle with Chicken in Basil Pesto and
Bell Pepper Coulis

Sausage and Broccoli Rabe Penne

Soft Polenta with Sliced Beef and Parmesan

Southeast Asian–Style Pasta Primavera

Beef Maki Roll

Chicken and Pumpkin Curry

Chicken Scaloppine with Linguine and Spinach

Chicken Stewed with Red Wine
and Wild Mushrooms

Barley "Risotto"

Chicken with Quinoa Tabbouleh

Orange-Cumin Glazed Pork Tenderloin

Pancetta-Wrapped Chicken Breast
with Pesto Orzo and Grilled Zucchini

Roast Chicken with Pasta Gratin

Kota Kapama (Cinnamon Chicken)

Stir-Fried Beef with Scallions and Mushrooms

Tiny Tacos

Superstuffed Steak Soft Taco

Acapulco-Style Mahi Mahi Ceviche

Alaskan Salmon in a Barley, Spring
Vegetables, and Port Reduction

Baked Asian-Style Salmon

Cape Cod Baked Scallops with Lime

Grilled Salmon with Vegetable Couscous
and Artichoke Vinaigrette

Grilled Tuna with Plum Salsa
and Boiled New Potatoes

Pan Roasted Halibut with Chickpeas
and Roasted Tomato Pasta

Poached Albacore Tuna with Pappardelle

Salmon and Edamame Penne

Salmon Baked in Paper

Scallops in Orange Sauce

Scampi

Shrimp with Israeli Couscous, Spring Peas,
Mint, and Lemon

Spicy Salmon Lettuce "Gyros"

Tilapia with Papaya Ginger Relish
and Summer Squash

Beef and Sun-Dried Tomato Flatbread Pizza

Naan Pizza with Canadian Bacon,
Asparagus, and Fontina Cheese

Triple Jump Pizza

Basque Grilled Vegetable Kebabs
with Key Lime Chimichurri

Curried Lentils with Butternut Squash

Eggplant Sandwich

Panini with Brie, Chocolate, and Olives

Tortilla Pie

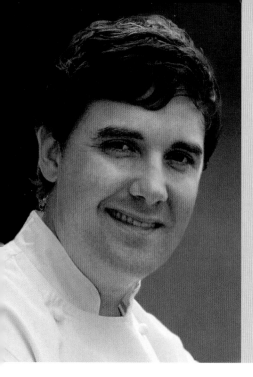

JOHN FRASER

John Fraser celebrates completing a marathon like many other runners do—with a bottle of wine (Silver Oak Cabernet) and something rich, such as this baked macaroni and cheese. "This dish is really supposed to be eaten after a long night out," says Fraser, who is the chef-owner of Dovetail in New York City. "But you could say running a marathon is similar." The California native earned a PR of 3:36 at his hometown race, the Los Angeles Marathon, in 2006, and during peak training logs 55 miles a week—sometimes when work finishes at 1 a.m. That helps explain why New York City is a favorite marathon, too. "I don't have time to take the weekend off," says Fraser, who has raced New York twice. "This way I can work on Saturday, run on Sunday, and be back at work on Monday." For more, go to dovetailnyc.com.

Baked Macaroni and Artisanal Cheese `RECOVERY` with Chorizo and Piquillo Peppers

"The artisanal Cheddar and pork chorizo make this really indulgent," John Fraser says, and a special treat. Jarred roasted piquillo peppers from Spain have a spicy-sweet flavor and can be found at specialty food shops. Use jarred roasted red peppers as a substitute. For more from John Fraser, see page 10.

Makes 4 servings

PREP TIME: 20 MINUTES / COOK TIME: 35–40 MINUTES

8 ounces macaroni, cooked al dente

4 tablespoons unsalted butter

¼ cup unbleached or all-purpose flour

1 cup 1% low-fat milk

2 cups grated artisanal Cheddar cheese

¼ teaspoon grated fresh nutmeg

Salt and white pepper to taste

¾ cup chorizo sausage, casing removed and diced

½ cup chopped basil, loosely packed

¼ cup piquillo peppers, julienned (optional)

¼ cup bread crumbs

2 tablespoons extra virgin olive oil

Preheat the oven to 325°F. Cook the macaroni to al dente according to package directions; set aside. Make a roux by heating the butter and flour in a large pot, stirring constantly on very low heat until blonde. Add the milk; simmer on medium-low heat for 10 to 15 minutes (the mixture will be thick). Add the cheese, slowly, whisking to make sure it melts all the way through. Add the nutmeg and season with the salt and white pepper, then fold in the cooked macaroni. Remove the pot from the heat and add the chorizo, basil, and peppers. Place in a 13″ x 9″ baking dish. Cover with the bread crumbs and drizzle the olive oil on top. Bake for 15 minutes or until done and the top is golden brown.

PER SERVING: 420 CALORIES • 16 G PROTEIN • 22 G CARBOHYDRATES • 30 G FAT

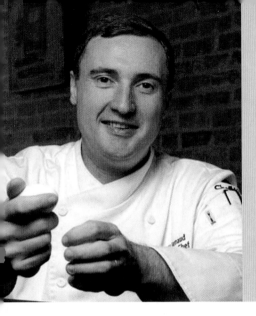

CYRIL RENAUD

A Frenchman without bread and butter is a Frenchman who can lose 30 pounds. At least, that's what Cyril Renaud concluded when he revamped his diet and exercise to drop weight after hitting a high of 205 pounds. "As much as I love bread and butter, I think cutting them out was the most effective thing I did," says the chef, whose restaurant Bar Breton in New York City showcases the cuisine of his native Brittany. That and running 4 or 5 miles daily, typically from his home in Brooklyn, over the Brooklyn Bridge and back. For more, go to chefpiano.com.

Brown Rice with Blood Oranges and Raisins

`QUICK AND EASY` `TRAINING`

Cyril Renaud says he likes this simple dish because it's "nice and clean, without too many flavors."

Blood oranges are rich in vitamin C, folate, and fiber. A whole grain, brown rice is a good source of carbs, with 46 grams in 1 cup cooked. One cup also provides 88 percent of the Daily Value for manganese, a mineral necessary for converting protein and carbohydrates into energy.

Makes 5 cups

PREP TIME: 10 MINUTES / COOK TIME: 40 MINUTES

3 blood oranges

½ cup raisins

2 tablespoons Dijon mustard

2 tablespoons sugar

2 tablespoons soy sauce

4 cups cooked long grain brown rice

Grate enough of 1 orange to get 2 teaspoons of peel. Squeeze 2 of the oranges to collect 1 cup of juice. Remove the segments from the third orange and set them aside for garnish.

Bring the juice to a boil in a small pot, remove from heat, and add the raisins to soak. Once the juice has cooled, add the peel, mustard, sugar, and soy sauce. Mix it into the cooked brown rice and garnish with orange segments.

PER SERVING: 341 CALORIES • 7 G PROTEIN • 76 G CARBOHYDRATES • 2 G FAT

Bucatini with Merguez Sausage

Spring peas are a rich source of vitamins, minerals, fiber, and protein. One cup of boiled peas provides more than half of the Daily Value of vitamin K, which is important for bone and cardiovascular health. For more from Daniel Humm, see page 144.

Makes 4 servings

PREP TIME: 15 MINUTES / COOK TIME: 45–55 MINUTES

2 tablespoons extra virgin olive oil

1 pound merguez sausage (or lamb sausage)

1 small onion, diced

2 cloves garlic, minced

1 cup dry white wine

1 can (14.5 ounces) whole, peeled tomatoes

Salt, to taste

1 pound bucatini (or spaghetti or other long, thin pasta)

$\frac{1}{2}$ cup frozen spring peas

Extra virgin olive oil, as needed to finish (optional)

1 bunch mint, without stems

Grated Pecorino cheese (optional)

Heat a large skillet with 1 tablespoon of olive oil. Remove the sausage from its casing and place in the heated skillet. While browning the sausage, break it up into small pieces with the back of a wooden spoon. Once browned, remove it from the pan and set it aside. Drain the fat from the pan. In the same pan, add the remaining tablespoon of olive oil and sauté the onions until golden, about 5 minutes. Add the white wine and cook until it's reduced by half. Add the cooked sausage and can of tomatoes, with juice, to the pan. Break up the tomatoes with a wooden spoon. Cook over low heat for 30 to 40 minutes to reduce the sauce.

In a 12-quart stockpot, bring water that has been liberally salted to a boil. Add the pasta and cook for about 6 to 7 minutes to desired doneness.

Add the peas to the tomato and sausage mixture. The peas will only take about 2 minutes to cook through. Season the sauce to taste with salt.

Drain the pasta into a colander, then add it to the pan with the sauce and toss to combine.

Turn the pasta out onto a large serving platter and finish with olive oil, mint leaves, and grated pecorino cheese.

PER SERVING (WITHOUT GRATED CHEESE AND ADDITIONAL OLIVE OIL):
796 CALORIES • 34 G PROTEIN • 95 G CARBOHYDRATES • 24 G FAT

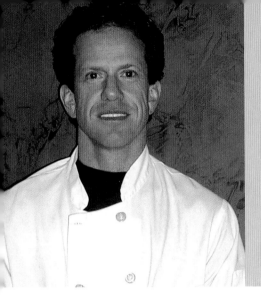

PAUL RAFTIS

Paul Raftis has pursued both cooking and running with equal gusto. He opened Paolo's Italian Restaurant in Kent, Washington, his hometown, nearly 2 decades ago, serving runner-friendly dishes packed with carbs and protein. He's also racked up 16 marathons, including Boston four times (with a PR of 3:17). "Back in junior high I was interested in a girl on the track team, so I gave running a try," Raftis says. "I discovered I actually liked running, so I stuck with it." For more, go to paolositalian.com.

Fettuccine Paolo

`TRAINING`

Paul Raftis likes to fuel up with this carb- and protein-filled dish before a big race. One medium artichoke provides 41 percent of the Daily Value for fiber and just 64 calories. Eating artichokes has also been linked with reductions in blood cholesterol levels. For more from Paul Raftis, see page 143.

Makes 2 servings

PREP TIME: 15 MINUTES / COOK TIME: 6 MINUTES

4 teaspoons extra virgin olive oil

1 red bell pepper, thinly sliced

1 teaspoon chopped garlic

1⅓ cups chicken stock

4 teaspoons balsamic vinegar

½ cup sun-dried tomatoes, sliced

½ cup marinated artichoke hearts with liquid

1½ cups sliced grilled chicken

2 tablespoons thinly sliced fresh basil

Salt and pepper, to taste

6 ounces fettuccine

2 teaspoons grated Parmesan cheese

Rehydrate the sun-dried tomatoes by placing them in a bowl with 1 cup warm water. Soak for 1 hour, or until softened. Gently squeeze to remove the excess liquid. Set aside.

Heat the olive oil over medium heat in a large skillet. Add the bell pepper and cook 3 minutes, or until soft. Add the garlic, and cook, stirring frequently, for 30 seconds. Add the stock and vinegar, bring to a boil, and simmer until reduced by half. Add the sun-dried tomatoes, artichoke hearts and liquid, grilled chicken, and basil. Season with salt and pepper. Keep warm. Cook the fettuccine according to package instructions. Drain the fettuccine, add to the pasta sauce, and mix thoroughly. Top with the Parmesan cheese.

PER SERVING: 580 CALORIES • 44 G PROTEIN • 66 G CARBOHYDRATES • 17 G FAT

GIANCARLA BODONI

Giancarla Bodoni's cooking career started with a paintbrush. To help pay for art school, she worked in a Miami café. There she met her husband, Pino, who had just opened a restaurant. More than a quarter century later, the two continue to helm Escopazzo, which means "going crazy," serving organic Italian food on Miami's South Beach. Bodoni, a former tennis player, gave up the sport for running—"with my schedule, I needed an activity I could do on my own," she says—she hasn't given up art. She painted a mural on one of the restaurant's walls depicting famous sites, such as the Roman Coliseum, inspired by the runs she takes when visiting family in Italy. For more, go to escopazzo.com.

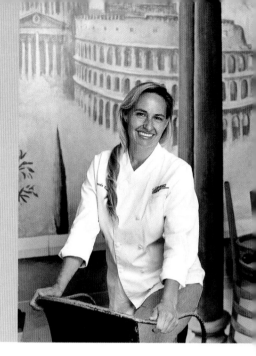

Linguine with Genovese Pesto

TRAINING

"With its range of pastas and proteins, Italian food is a natural for runners," Giancarla Bodoni says. She especially likes this linguine pesto because of the energizing carbs from the pasta, the muscle-building protein from the pine nuts, and the heart-healthy fats from the olive oil. A good source of vitamin C, garlic has antibacterial and cholesterol-lowering properties and can reduce the inflammation caused by exercise. For more from Giancarla Bodoni, see page 73.

Makes 6 servings

PREP TIME: 15 MINUTES / COOK TIME: 11 MINUTES

¾ cup extra virgin olive oil

½ cup pine nuts

2 garlic cloves

½ teaspoon salt

5 cups fresh basil leaves, stems removed

⅓ cup grated Parmesan cheese

1 pound linguine

1 potato, peeled and diced into ½" pieces

2 cups string beans, trimmed and halved

Salt to taste

(continued)

Place the olive oil, pine nuts, garlic, and salt in a blender and process. Keep the blender at high speed, and pulse as you add the basil leaves. Push the leaves onto the blade with a rubber spatula. Try to blend all of the basil as quickly as possible so as not to create too much heat. Process until smooth. Add the cheese. Makes about 2 cups of pesto sauce.

In a 4- to 6-quart pot, add the linguine to boiling, salted water. After 5 minutes, add the diced potato and beans. Finish cooking the linguine according to package directions. Add the salt.

Drain the water, reserving about $1/2$ cup. Place the pasta and vegetables back in the pot and add the pesto (do not reheat pot). Mix well, adding a little of the pasta water if necessary. Add more grated cheese to taste.

PER SERVING: 659 CALORIES • 15 G PROTEIN • 64 G CARBOHYDRATES • 38 G FAT

Marathon Fettuccine in Charred Tomato Sauce and Shrimp

Bobby Flay made this prerace meal with American Olympic marathoner Deena Kastor, who loves to cook. The two cooked together at Flay's New York City restaurant Bar Americain a few months before they both ran the 2006 New York City Marathon. For more from Bobby Flay, see page 149.

Makes 4 servings

PREP TIME: 15 MINUTES / COOK TIME: 50 MINUTES

Charred Tomatoes

12 plum tomatoes

2 tablespoons olive oil

Salt and pepper to taste

Sauce

2 tablespoons extra-virgin olive oil

1 medium Spanish onion, finely chopped

2 cloves garlic, thinly sliced

1/2 teaspoon crushed red-pepper flakes

Salt and freshly ground black pepper to taste

3 tablespoons coarsely chopped fresh basil

3/4 pound fresh fettuccine, cooked al dente

Fresh basil sprigs, for garnish

Shrimp

2 tablespoons extra-virgin olive oil

Salt and freshly ground black pepper

20 large shrimp, peeled and deveined

Tomatoes

Preheat broiler or grill pan over high heat. Brush tomatoes with oil and season with salt and pepper.

If using a broiler: Put the tomatoes on a sheet pan and place them under the broiler (about 4″ from the direct heat) until charred on all sides, turning several times with tongs, about 10 to 12 minutes.

If using a grill pan: Place the tomatoes on a very hot grill pan and char on all sides, turning with tongs, about 7 to 10 minutes.

Remove them from the oven, let them cool slightly, and coarsely chop.

(continued on page 89)

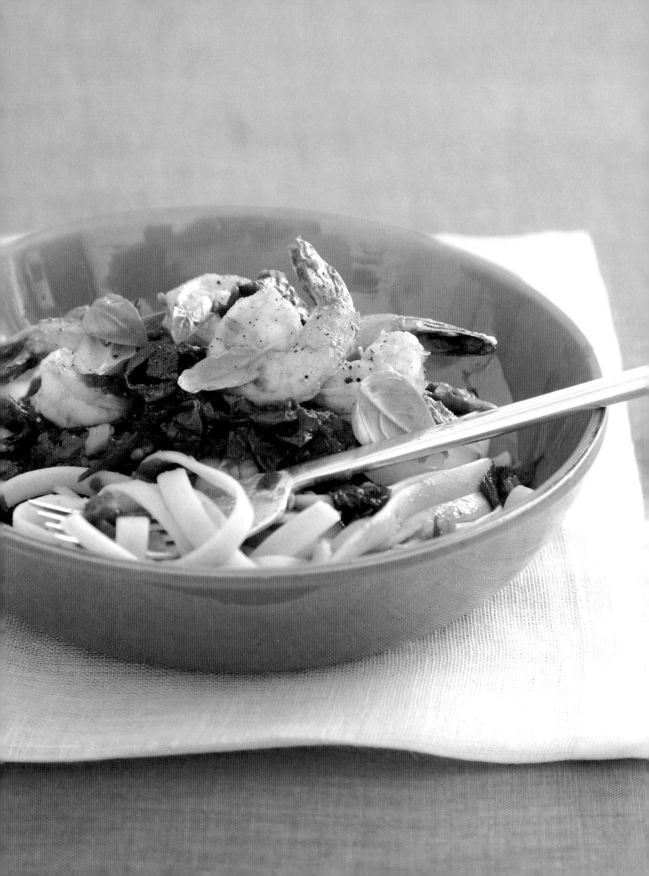

Sauce

Heat the oil in a large, high-sided sauté pan over medium-high heat. Add the onion and cook until soft, 2 to 3 minutes. Add the garlic and red-pepper flakes and cook for 30 seconds.

Add the charred tomatoes, salt, and pepper and cook until the tomatoes are soft and break down completely, 20 to 30 minutes. Stir in the basil. Add the cooked pasta and, using tongs, stir to coat the pasta evenly.

Divide the pasta among four large, shallow bowls and top with 5 of the pan-sautéed shrimp (instructions below). Garnish with the basil sprigs.

Shrimp

Heat the oil in a large, nonstick sauté pan over medium-high heat until shimmering. Season the shrimp with salt and pepper and cook, stirring frequently, until the shrimp is lightly golden-brown on both sides and just cooked through, 1 to 2 minutes per side.

PER SERVING: 512 CALORIES • 19 G PROTEIN • 58 G CARBOHYDRATES • 24 G FAT

Vincent's Mushroom Risotto

 TRAINING

One cup of cooked arborio, a short-grain Italian rice used to make risotto, provides more than 53 grams of carbohydrates. For more from Vincent Francoual, see pages 62, 142, and 188.

see pages 62, 142, and 188.

Makes 10 servings

PREP TIME: 20 MINUTES / COOK TIME: 50 MINUTES

Risotto

2½–3 quarts low-sodium vegetable broth (or use homemade, if desired)

1 sprig each fresh thyme and fresh rosemary, for bouquet garni

2 cloves garlic, for bouquet garni

1 medium yellow onion, diced

8 tablespoons unsalted butter (1 stick)

1 pound arborio rice

½ cup white wine

1 cup grated Parmesan cheese

½ cup mascarpone cheese

In a large pot, bring the vegetable broth to a simmer over medium heat. Keep warm on the stove.

To make the bouquet garni, bundle a cheesecloth square around the rosemary, thyme, and garlic. Tie pouch with string. Melt 4 tablespoons of the butter in a medium skillet over medium-high heat, add the onion, and cook, stirring frequently, for 3 minutes. Add the rice and the bouquet garni, and cook and stir well for 1 minute, until all rice grains are coated. Add the wine and continue stirring for another minute or 2. Add a ladle of hot vegetable stock and stir until the broth is absorbed. Repeat this until the rice is just cooked al dente. Remove the bouquet garni and add the remaining 4 tablespoons of butter and stir. Add the Parmesan and mascarpone cheeses. Stir until cheese is melted.

Ladle into 1 large bowl or individual serving dishes.

Garnish for risotto

½ cup chopped oven-dried or sun-dried tomatoes

1 cup sautéed mushrooms (shitake, oyster, or cremini)

1 cup diced butternut squash, steamed

Salt and pepper to taste

Olive oil or walnut oil

Garnish the serving dish with the mushrooms, tomatoes, and butternut squash. Season with salt and pepper. Drizzle olive oil or walnut oil on the rice.

PER SERVING: 424 CALORIES • 9 G PROTEIN • 44 G CARBOHYDRATES • 22 G FAT

Orecchiette Carbonara with Chicken and Broccoli

Orecchiette—from the Italian orecchio, *or ear—are small, ear-shaped pasta. The shape makes them ideal for holding sauces. For more from James Dangler, see pages 96 and 101.*

Makes 4 servings

PREP TIME: 15 MINUTES / COOK TIME: 18–20 MINUTES, INCLUDING COOKING THE PASTA

1 pound orecchiette

1 boneless, skinless chicken breast, cut into 1" cubes (about 6 ounces)

1 tablespoon extra virgin olive oil

3 cloves garlic, chopped

1 large shallot, chopped

½ cup chopped red or yellow bell pepper

¼ cup chopped onion

¼ cup sliced portobello mushrooms (or your favorite mushrooms)

1 tablespoon sun-dried tomatoes, julienned (about 1 piece)

5–6 medium asparagus, trimmed and cut into 1" pieces

2 cups broccoli florets

Salt and pepper to taste

1 pint half-and-half

1 tablespoon crisply cooked pancetta or bacon (about ½ slice pancetta or 1 slice bacon)

Chopped fresh basil, thyme, and oregano to taste

Grated Parmesan cheese to taste

Cook the orecchiette according to package directions. Set aside.

Sauté the chicken breast in olive oil in a large skillet until almost cooked through, about 2 to 3 minutes. Add the garlic, shallots, peppers, onion, mushrooms, sun-dried tomatoes, asparagus, and broccoli florets. Continue cooking until the vegetables are al dente and the chicken is completely cooked through, about 5 to 7 minutes. Add salt and pepper to taste.

Add the half-and-half to the pan and bring to a slow simmer on medium heat. Cook until the mixture is slightly thickened, about 2 to 3 minutes, and remove the pan from the heat.

Drop the cooked pasta into simmering water for 1 minute. Drain the pasta. Toss the pasta with the chicken and vegetables in cream sauce. Divide among 4 pasta bowls and top with the pancetta or bacon, herbs, and cheese to taste.

PER SERVING: 699 CALORIES, 33 G PROTEIN, 99 G CARBOHYDRATES, 20 G FAT

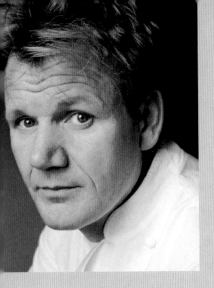

GORDON RAMSAY

Gordon Ramsay, one of only a few British chefs to be awarded three stars by the prestigious Michelin Guide, keeps it simple when it comes to fueling for a big race. "The night before a marathon is about loading up on carbs, not making complicated dishes," says the chef, whose fiery personality lights up such reality TV cooking shows as *Hell's Kitchen* and *Kitchen Nightmares*. His training routine is also simple: A few nights a week he runs 10 miles home from his London restaurant, wearing a weighted backpack. A regular at the London Marathon (with a PR of 3:35), Ramsay has finished South Africa's 54-mile Comrades ultramarathon three times. His cooking career is equally impressive, with more than a dozen each restaurants and cookbooks. Although he avoids fatty foods before a race, Ramsay does like to tuck into barbecue afterward. "That and a good, hot soak." For more, go to gordonramsay.com.

Pancetta Spaghetti

QUICK AND EASY   TRAINING

"This pasta is easy to make and has great flavor without using cream or butter," Gordon Ramsay says. Garlic improves circulation by dilating blood vessels and improving blood flow. It also reduces the inflammation that can come with joint pain and is a good source of vitamin C.

Makes 2 hearty servings

PREP TIME: 10 MINUTES + 1 HOUR TO INFUSE GARLIC OIL / COOK TIME: 15 MINUTES

½ cup extra virgin olive oil

5 cloves garlic, finely sliced

8 ounces spaghetti

4 ounces finely diced pancetta

¼ cup flat-leaf parsley, chopped and loosely packed

To make garlic oil, heat the olive oil in a small saucepan over medium heat and add the garlic. Remove it from the stove and let it infuse for 1 hour, then discard the garlic. Cook the pasta according to package directions. Add 2 tablespoons of the garlic oil to a separate pan and fry the pancetta until cooked (about 3 to 4 minutes).

Drain the pasta and add it to the pancetta. Garnish the pasta with the parsley.

PER SERVING: 600 CALORIES • 10 G PROTEIN • 80 G CARBOHYDRATES • 22 G FAT

JOËL ANTUNES

Like many runners, Joël Antunes obsesses over carbs in the weeks leading up to a big event. "I incorporate pasta into my diet once a day 2 weeks before a race," says the French-born chef. He prepared and enjoyed this Pasta Mediterranée multiple times before completing the challenging 2005 Biathlon du Sancy, a 10-mile run and 40-mile mountain bike race in France's mountainous Massif Central region, where he placed seventh. Since leaving his eponymous restaurant Joël Brasserie in Atlanta to refashion New York City's iconic Oak Room, Antunes has been spending time traveling the world.

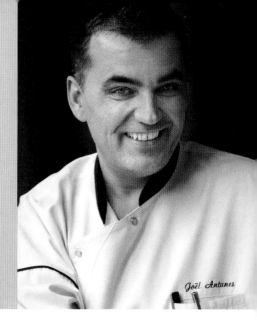

Pasta Mediterranée

QUICK AND EASY / TRAINING

This pasta dish swaps fat for flavor. "I like light, Mediterranean dishes that use little cream or butter," says Joël Antunes. The eggplant, zucchini, and tomatoes provide potassium and vitamin C.

Makes 2 servings

PREP TIME: 10 MINUTES / COOK TIME: 12–15 MINUTES

8 ounces penne pasta

2 tablespoons extra virgin olive oil + additional oil to taste

¼ cup sun-dried tomatoes in oil, drained

¼ cup diced eggplant

¼ cup diced zucchini

2 tablespoons grated Parmesan cheese

½ cup mozzarella cubes

5 leaves fresh basil, chopped

Sea salt and freshly ground pepper to taste

Boil the pasta for 5 minutes or according to package directions. Drain. Heat 1 tablespoon of olive oil in a large skillet over medium-high heat. Add the tomatoes, eggplant, and zucchini and cook, stirring frequently, for 4 minutes. Remove from the heat. Add the pasta and vegetables to a large skillet and cook in the remaining tablespoon of olive oil for 3 minutes, then remove from the heat. Mix in the Parmesan and mozzarella cheeses and basil. Season with sea salt, freshly ground black pepper, and more olive oil to taste.

PER SERVING: 670 CALORIES • 25 G PROTEIN • 88 G CARBOHYDRATES • 24 G FAT

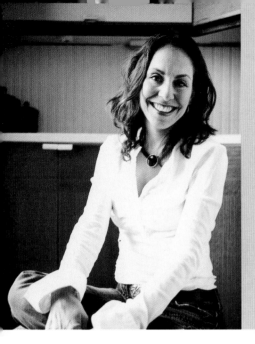

GRACE PARISI

A funny thing happened when Grace Parisi began racing half and full marathons. "Once I hit 40, I started placing in my age group, which took the sting off of being 40," says the New York City–based author of the cookbook *Get Saucy*. Eventually she qualified for and ran the Boston Marathon, finishing in 3:56. The senior recipe developer for *Food & Wine* magazine creates and tests 40 to 60 recipes every month. "I run to counteract the effects of eating and cooking all day," says Parisi, who averages about 25 miles weekly and helped start a women's running club called Brooklyn Queens Excel, or BQE, a reference to the New York City highway with the same initials. For more, go to foodandwine.com.

Penne Arrabbiata

`TRAINING`

Cooked tomatoes are an excellent source of lycopene, an antioxidant that helps protect against cancer and benefits cardiovascular and eye health. For more from Grace Parisi, see page 121.

Makes 4 servings

PREP TIME: 10 MINUTES / COOK TIME: 30 MINUTES

1 tablespoon extra virgin olive oil	28 ounces diced or petite-cut tomatoes
4 ounces pancetta or bacon, finely diced	Pinch of sugar
1/2 small onion, minced	Salt and freshly ground pepper to taste
1 large garlic clove, minced	12 ounces penne
1/2 teaspoon crushed red-pepper flakes	Parmigiano-Reggiano cheese, freshly grated

Heat the oil in a large saucepan over medium-high heat. Add the pancetta, onion, and garlic. Cook, stirring occasionally, until the pancetta just begins to turn pink and the onion is golden, about 5 minutes. Add the crushed red pepper and cook until the pancetta starts to brown. Add the tomatoes with their juices and sugar. Season with the salt and pepper and bring to a boil. Reduce the heat to medium-low, and cook, partially covered, until the sauce is thickened, about 30 minutes. Meanwhile, cook the penne in plenty of salted water until it's al dente, about 7 to 9 minutes. Drain and return it to the pot. Add half of the sauce and cook, stirring, for 1 minute. Spoon the penne into bowls, serving the remaining sauce and the grated cheese on top.

PER SERVING: 508 CALORIES • 20 G PROTEIN • 71 G CARBOHYDRATES • 15 G FAT

JOE BASTIANICH

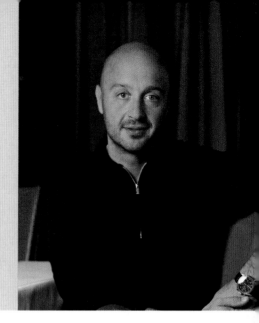

Good food and wine are abundant when you own 18 Italian restaurants, which helps explain why Joe Bastianich had hit 245 pounds. "I was on doctor's orders to lose weight," says the restaurateur and winemaker. While he is still able to enjoy the Italian food he and his chef-partners Mario Batali and Lidia Bastianich (his mom) helped make famous, he began practicing portion control, avoiding late-night eating, and focusing on healthier dishes. Taking a year to train for the 2008 New York City Marathon, Bastianich dropped 45 pounds and finished in 3:46. For more, go to bastianich.com.

Rigatoni with Early Asparagus and Shiitake Mushrooms

`TRAINING`

For a dose of carbs, Joe Bastianich loves simple, healthy pasta dishes made with just a bit of olive oil and plenty of vegetables. For more from Joe Bastianich, see page 193.

Makes 6 servings

PREP TIME: 10 MINUTES / COOK TIME: 15–20 MINUTES

1 pound rigatoni

5 tablespoons extra virgin olive oil

3 cloves garlic, thinly sliced

¾ pound shiitake mushrooms, sliced

Salt and pepper to taste

½ pound asparagus, cut into 1" pieces

2 tablespoons chopped fresh parsley

2 tablespoons grated lemon peel

¼ cup grated Parmigiano Reggiano cheese

In a large pot, cook the pasta according to package directions; drain, reserving 1 cup of pasta water. Heat 3 tablespoons of the olive oil in a large saucepan over medium-high heat. Add the garlic and cook, stirring frequently, until it begins to turn gold. Add the mushrooms. Season the garlic-mushroom mixture with the salt and pepper. Cook the mushrooms, stirring frequently, until darkened, about 5 minutes. Add the asparagus and toss gently to coat. Turn the heat under the saucepan to high and add 1 cup of the reserved pasta water. Cook until the water reduces by half, about 30 seconds. Add the cooked, drained pasta to the skillet. Toss over high heat for 1 minute. Turn off heat and toss with parsley, grated lemon peel, and cheese. Drizzle with the remaining 2 tablespoons of olive oil and serve.

PER SERVING: 440 CALORIES • 12 G PROTEIN • 65 G CARBOHYDRATES • 14 G FAT

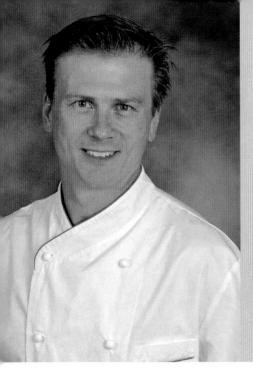

JAMES DANGLER

James Dangler credits marathon training with saving his life. On the morning of September 11, 2001, the chef was working at Roy's New York in lower Manhattan, one block from the World Trade Center. At first he thought nothing of the electricity going off and on. But then glass started shattering, and by the time he left the building, debris was raining down. "I couldn't believe the inferno I saw, just a baseball-throw away," says Dangler, who is originally from Rochester, New York. "I turned and ran like hell." Now Dangler, who is executive chef at the Ritz-Carlton Westchester in White Plains, New York, finds that races he does in the city are more meaningful. He's run the New York City Marathon four times, and his PR of 2:55 is nearly an hour faster than his first finish 14 years earlier. For more, go to ritzcarlton.com.

Rotelle with Chicken in Basil Pesto and Bell Pepper Coulis

`TRAINING`

This spin on the usual pasta-and-protein combination uses roasted red peppers instead of marinara sauce. Two tablespoons of pesto, made with olive oil and pine nuts, contain 7 grams of heart-healthy monounsaturated fat. For more from James Dangler, see pages 91 and 101.

Makes 4 servings

PREP TIME: 25 MINUTES / COOK TIME: 16–20 MINUTES

Pesto

5 ounces fresh basil

3 cloves garlic

2 tablespoons pine nuts, toasted

1/4 cup grated Parmesan cheese

1/2 cup extra-virgin olive oil

Bell Pepper Coulis

1 jar (12 ounces) roasted red peppers, drained

1/4 cup water

1 tablespoon dark balsamic vinegar

1 teaspoon jarred, grated horseradish

Pinch of sugar

Salt and pepper to taste

Chicken and Pasta

4 chicken breasts (about 2½ pounds), cut into pieces or strips

2 tablespoons extra virgin olive oil

2 cloves garlic, minced

¾ cup white wine

1 pound rotelle

1 tablespoon toasted pine nuts

1 tablespoon basil, sliced into thin strips

2 tablespoons grated Parmesan cheese

Pesto

Place basil, garlic, pine nuts, Parmesan, and olive oil in a food processor and puree.

Bell Pepper Coulis

Puree red pepper, water, balsamic vinegar, horseradish, sugar, and salt and pepper in a blender. Warm the mixture in a saucepan. Remove from heat and place in 4 pasta bowls.

Chicken and Pasta

Season the chicken with salt and pepper. Heat the oil in a skillet. Add the chicken and minced garlic and cook through, about 8 to 10 minutes on each side. Add the white wine, scraping the pan to loosen any brown bits. Simmer to reduce the liquid by half. Add 5 tablespoons of the pesto and mix together. Cook the pasta according to the package directions, drain, and toss the pasta with the sauce. Add the toasted pine nuts, basil, and grated Parmesan. Place the pasta into the bowl over the bell-pepper coulis.

PER SERVING: 760 CALORIES • 46 G PROTEIN • 92 G CARBOHYDRATES • 19 G FAT

Sausage and Broccoli Rabe Penne TRAINING

Pam Anderson calls this recipe "the perfect one-dish pasta" because it contains a mix of protein, vegetables, and carbohydrates. Broccoli rabe, a dark leafy green, is more closely related to kale than broccoli and is a good source of fiber, calcium, iron, and phytochemical antioxidants. For more from Pam Anderson, see pages 30 and 152.

Makes 6 servings

PREP TIME: 15 MINUTES/COOK TIME: 35 MINUTES

12 ounces lean Italian turkey sausage

3 tablespoons extra virgin olive oil

1/4 cup + 1 quart water

1/2 cup pitted oil-cured olives, coarsely chopped

3 peeled garlic cloves, minced

1/2 teaspoon red-pepper flakes

1 can (28 ounces) crushed tomatoes

3/4 teaspoon salt

12 ounces penne

8 cups coarsely chopped broccoli rabe (about 1/2 bunch)

1/2 cup crumbled feta cheese

Bring the sausage, olive oil, and water to simmer in a large covered pot over medium-high heat. Cook until the water evaporates, about 5 minutes. Uncover and fry the sausage, turning frequently, until well browned, a couple of minutes longer. Remove the sausage, cool slightly, and slice in 1/2" rounds.

Add the olives, garlic, and pepper flakes to the empty pot. When the garlic starts to turn golden, stir in the tomatoes and sausages when ready. Continue to simmer, partially covered, until the flavors meld, about 10 minutes. Add 1 quart of water and the salt to the sauce; bring to a boil. Add the penne and cook partially covered for 10 minutes. Add the broccoli rabe; cook, partially covered and stirring occasionally, until pasta and broccoli rabe are tender, about 5 more minutes. Serve, topping each portion with crumbled feta.

PER SERVING: 527 CALORIES, 23 G PROTEIN, 60 G CARBOHYDRATES, 23 G FAT

Soft Polenta with Sliced Beef and Parmesan

An Italian staple made from cornmeal, polenta is a good source of carbohydrates, with 26 grams per half-cup serving. Look for whole grain polenta instead of "degerminated" polenta, which has a longer shelf life but fewer nutrients. Cooked tomatoes are an excellent source of lycopene, which has been shown to fight cancer and cardiovascular disease and to benefit eye health. Tomatoes also contain vitamin C, folate, and potassium. You can substitute 3 cups jarred tomato sauce. For more from Claude Solliard, see page 48.

Makes 6 first-course servings

PREP TIME: 30 MINUTES / COOK TIME: 1 HOUR 30 MINUTES

Tomato Sauce

- 1 tablespoon extra virgin olive oil
- 4 large garlic cloves, finely chopped
- 1 small onion, finely chopped
- 4 medium tomatoes, peeled, seeded, and chopped
- 2 cups canned tomato juice
- 1/8 teaspoon dried oregano
- 4 fresh basil leaves, rinsed and dried
- Kosher salt and freshly ground black pepper to taste

Polenta

- 4 teaspoons unsalted butter
- 2 garlic cloves, finely chopped
- 4 cups 2% low-fat milk + more as needed
- 2 cups instant polenta
- Salt and freshly ground black pepper to taste
- 1 cup grated or shaved Parmesan cheese

Beef

- 2 tablespoons extra-virgin olive oil
- 1 1/2 pounds sliced beef sirloin (about 2" to 3" long and 3/4" wide)
- 1 garlic clove, minced
- 1 tablespoon finely chopped flat-leaf parsley

Tomato Sauce

Warm the olive oil in a medium saucepan over moderate heat. Add the garlic and onion and cook, stirring frequently, until the onion is golden, about 5 minutes. Add the tomatoes and tomato juice, stirring to combine. Lower the heat and cook, uncovered, until the mixture has thickened and the tomatoes have dissolved into the sauce, about 1 hour. Stir in the oregano, basil, salt, and pepper, and keep the sauce warm.

Makes about 3 cups

(continued)

Polenta

Melt the butter until foamy over moderate heat in a medium pan. Add the garlic and cook, stirring frequently, until garlic is lightly colored, about 3 minutes. Add milk and bring to a boil. Slowly add polenta and cook, stirring constantly, until the liquids have been absorbed, about 5 to 8 minutes. Add the salt and pepper and keep the polenta warm.

Beef

Add the olive oil to a medium sauté pan over moderate heat. When the oil is hot, add the beef and sauté until it is lightly colored, for about 3 minutes. Add the garlic and prepared tomato sauce and cook for about 2 minutes.

Spoon the polenta into the center of 6 soup plates. (If the polenta has thickened, use warm milk to thin the consistency). Arrange the beef and tomato sauce equally over the polenta and sprinkle with chopped parsley and shaved Parmesan.

PER SERVING: 670 CALORIES • 47 G PROTEIN • 58 G CARBOHYDRATES • 28 G FAT

Southeast Asian–Style
Pasta Primavera

This pasta primavera is flavored with aromatic, floral kaffir lime leaves and lemongrass, staples in Southeast Asian cuisines, particularly Thai. Fresh kaffir lime leaves are used like bay leaves; cook with them but then remove before serving. Find them at Asian groceries or gourmet markets.

Colorful bell peppers are loaded with vitamins C and A. One cup of raw, sliced bell pepper provides almost 300 percent and more than 100 percent of the Daily Value for each, respectively. For more from James Dangler, see pages 91 and 96.

Makes 6 servings

PREP TIME: 20 MINUTES / COOK TIME: 15 MINUTES

8 ounces fettuccine or linguine
 (or any style Asian noodle,
 such as ramen, soba, or udon)
1 tablespoon extra virgin olive oil
1 teaspoon minced ginger
1 teaspoon minced garlic
1 teaspoon finely chopped lemongrass
1 kaffir lime leaf
1 cup julienned carrots
1 cup chopped shiitake mushrooms

½ cup chopped yellow bell peppers
½ cup chopped red bell peppers
10 asparagus tips
½ cup mung bean sprouts
1 tablespoon sesame oil
Salt and pepper to taste
Soy sauce to taste
1 tablespoon freshly squeezed lemon juice
Fresh basil or cilantro leaves to taste for
 garnish

Cook the pasta according to the package directions and set aside. Heat the olive oil in a large skillet or wok over medium-high heat. Add the ginger, garlic, lemon grass, and kaffir lime leaf. Cook for 1 minute or until fragrant.

Add carrots, mushrooms, bell peppers, and asparagus, and cook and stir for 3 to 4 minutes. Add the mung bean sprouts and cooked fettuccine and toss while continuing to cook. Drizzle with the sesame oil, soy sauce, and lemon juice and toss for another minute. Season with salt and pepper. Top with basil or cilantro and serve immediately.

PER SERVING: 277 CALORIES • 9 G PROTEIN • 38 G CARBOHYDRATES • 11 G FAT

Beef Maki Roll

Nori is seaweed dried into a sheet. It is a good source of protein as well as vitamins A, B₁, B₂, and C. You'll need a bamboo mat for rolling the sushi, available at Asian or gourmet markets. For more from Paul Muller, see page 77.

Makes 1 serving

PREP TIME: 45 MINUTES / COOK TIME: 20 MINUTES

1 cup Japanese short-grain rice

4–6 tablespoons seasoned sushi rice
vinegar + additional for vinegar water

1 sheet nori (dried seaweed wrap)

2 ounces prime beef (strip or ribeye),
grilled, chilled, and sliced into 6 bias cuts

Pinch of wasabi powder

½ tablespoon wasabi mayo

1 tablespoon shiitake mushrooms, grilled
and sliced

2 tablespoons finely chopped regular
arugula

1 tablespoon sliced chives

⅛ teaspoon Sriracha chili sauce for garnish

1 tablespoon pickled ginger

1 teaspoon wasabi paste

Sushi rice

Rinse the rice in cold running water 3 times.

Cook the rice in 1 cup of water, following package directions. Let cool.

Place the cooked rice in a bowl. Evenly distribute 4 to 6 tablespoons of seasoned sushi rice vinegar over the cooked rice, using a spatula to fold them together. When thoroughly mixed, the rice will be sticky. Cover and set aside.

To make the vinegar water, mix 5 parts water with 1 part rice vinegar. Set aside until ready to use.

Beef Maki Roll

Place the nori sheet on the bamboo mat.

Dip your hands in the vinegar water and scoop up a heaping handful of cooked and seasoned rice. (You will have rice left over.) Carefully spread the rice evenly over the nori to cover, leaving about ⅛″ of both long ends of the nori uncovered. Press lightly and then gently lift the nori and turn it over so that the rice side is directly on top of the bamboo mat, and press lightly again. (This means that the resulting roll has the rice on the outside.) Make sure you line the long edge of the nori up with the edge of the bamboo mat.

Arrange the cut beef from left to right on the nori, followed by the mushrooms and arugula.

Spread wasabi mayo, shiitake mushrooms, and arugula evenly from left to right.

Slowly roll up the filled nori from the bottom to the top to form a tube, using the bamboo mat, As you roll, squeeze the bamboo mat so that the roll is tight and the contents stay inside. Use just a little of the vinegar water to seal the edges of the roll together.

Remove the roll from the bamboo mat and let it rest for a couple of minutes on a cutting board. Then with a very sharp knife dipped in vinegar water, slice the roll into 8 to 10 evenly sized pieces.

Places the sliced roll on a plate and garnish with sriracha, pickled ginger, and wasabi paste.

PER SERVING: 450 CALORIES • 17 G PROTEIN • 62 G CARBOHYDRATES • 13 G FAT

Chicken and Pumpkin Curry

RECOVERY

"This is a very warming dish, perfect for cooler weather," says Patricia Wells. "It is influenced by a trip to Vietnam." You can substitute butternut squash for the pumpkin, if desired; both are good sources of vitamin A. Compounds in ginger fight the inflammation associated with joint pain and have been shown to combat some types of cancer. Turmeric, a spice included in curry powder mixes, has been found to be effective in preventing cancer and alleviating symptoms of arthritis. It has also been associated with slowing the progression of Alzheimer's disease. For more from Patricia Wells, see pages 16, 50, 181, and 194.

Makes 6 servings

PREP TIME: 20 MINUTES / COOK TIME: 15–20 MINUTES

Marinade

2 tablespoons minced fresh lemongrass

1 small red chili, seeded and chopped

3 tablespoons minced fresh ginger

2 tablespoons curry powder

Chicken

2 pounds boneless, skinless, chicken breasts, cubed

1 onion, halved and thinly sliced

3 cloves garlic, minced

1 tablespoon curry powder

1 small red chili, seeded and chopped

1 stalk lemongrass, peeled and bruised

1 teaspoon fine sea salt

1 teaspoon freshly ground black pepper

1 tablespoon sugar

⅓ cup coconut milk

¾ pound (about 3–4 cups) cubed fresh pumpkin

Marinade

Combine the lemongrass, chili, ginger, and curry powder in a small bowl. Place the cubed chicken in a zip-top bag and add the marinade ingredients. Mix to blend. Refrigerate for 1 hour or up to 4 hours.

Chicken

Combine the onion, garlic, curry powder, chili, and lemongrass, and cook, covered, over low heat until soft and translucent, about 3 minutes. Drain off the marinade and add the chicken, salt, pepper, and sugar, and cook for 2 minutes more. Add the coconut milk and simmer for 1 minute more. (You will find the mixture dry at this point, but it moistens as it cooks.) Add the cubed pumpkin and simmer, covered, until the chicken and pumpkin are cooked through, about 10 to 15 minutes. Remove from the heat and discard the lemongrass. Serve warm.

PER SERVING: 250 CALORIES • 32 G PROTEIN • 15 G CARBOHYDRATES • 7 G FAT

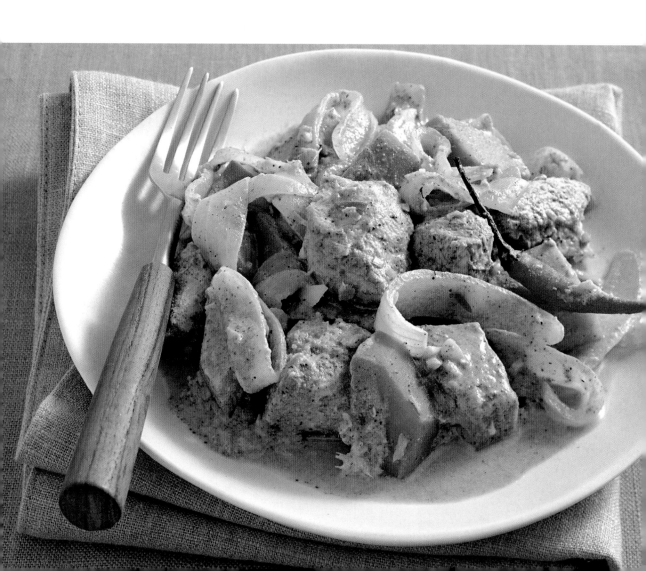

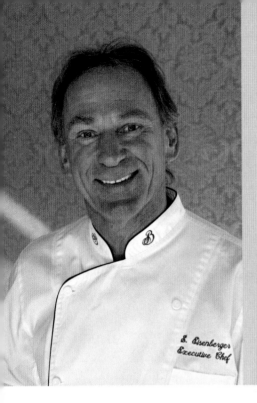

SIEGFRIED EISENBERGER

Running hills is not part of Siegfried Eisenberger's training program; it *is* his training program. The executive chef at the Broadmoor, a 3,000-acre resort in Colorado Springs, makes the most of the mountainous region by charging up hills on all of his four weekly runs. He trains on roads, trails, and stairs that ascend 1,200 feet for a single purpose—to run the Pikes Peak Ascent and Marathon, which consists of two events: a half-marathon that climbs nearly 8,000 feet to the peak on the first day, and a round-trip marathon—up and back down—on the following day. Eisenberger first ran the Ascent in 2001 when he was 53 and has run it every August since (with a PR of 3:45), doing both the Ascent and the marathon in the same weekend three times. "This race is great," says the Austrian native. "It reminds me that age is only a number." For more, go to broadmoor.com.

Chicken Scaloppine with Linguine and Spinach

`TRAINING`

The night before a morning run, Siegfried Eisenberger cooks a light dinner, such as this chicken and pasta dish. Chicken provides plenty of protein; one 5-ounce breast contains 35 grams, or 65 percent of the Daily Value for protein. Rich in cooked tomatoes, the antioxidant lycopene has been linked to a reduced incidence of some cancers, heart disease, and macular degeneration.

Makes 4 servings

PREP TIME: 30 MINUTES / COOK TIME: 40 MINUTES

8 ounces whole wheat linguine

4 skinless, boneless chicken breasts (about 5 ounces each)

Salt and pepper to taste

1 teaspoon chopped fresh thyme

2 tablespoons extra virgin olive oil

2 cloves garlic, finely chopped

6 ounces (about 3 cups) packaged baby spinach

1 teaspoon chopped fresh basil

1½ cups Broadmoor Tomato Sauce (recipe page 108)

1 tablespoon chopped fresh, flat-leaf parsley

½ cup grated Parmigiano-Reggiano cheese

(continued on page 108)

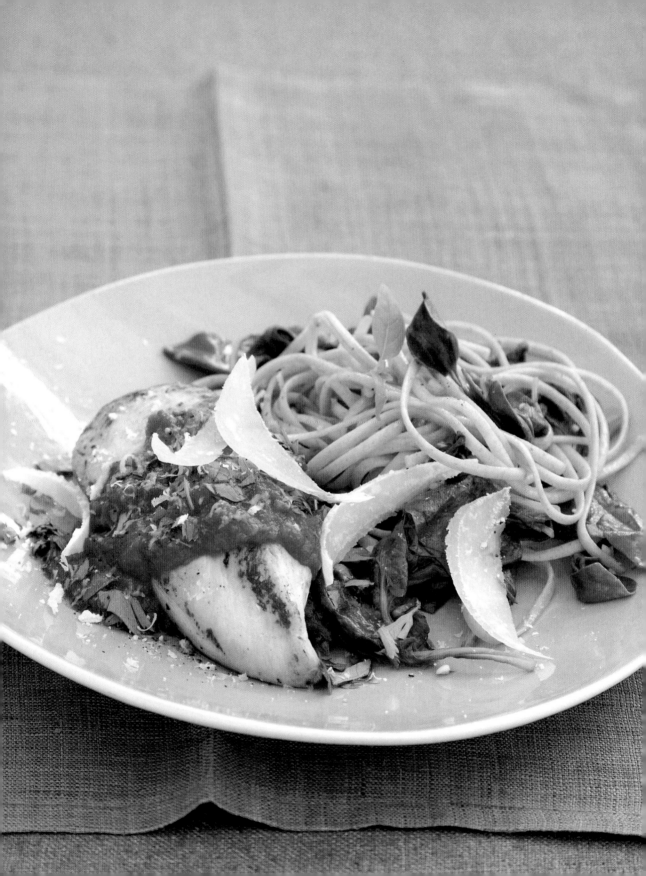

Cook the pasta according to package directions. Drain and set aside. Season the chicken with the salt, pepper, and thyme. Preheat a nonstick sauté skillet on medium-high heat. Brown the chicken on both sides and cook until done (about 7 minutes each side). Remove it from pan. Heat the olive oil in the skillet over high heat. Add the garlic, spinach, and basil and cook, stirring frequently for 5 minutes, or until fragrant. Add the pasta to the skillet, combining the pasta with the spinach mixture. Remove the skillet from the heat. Place in a serving dish, and top with the warm tomato sauce and sliced chicken breasts. Garnish with the parsley and cheese.

PER SERVING: 520 CALORIES • 46 G PROTEIN • 54 G CARBOHYDRATES • 15 G FAT

Broadmoor Tomato Sauce

Makes 1½ cups

1 tablespoon extra virgin olive oil

1 shallot, finely chopped

2 cloves garlic, minced

1 cup canned crushed tomatoes with liquid

½ cup tomato puree

1 tablespoon coarsely chopped fresh basil

1 teaspoon chopped fresh oregano

Salt and pepper to taste

Heat the olive oil in a large saucepan over medium heat. Add the shallot and garlic and cook, stirring frequently, for 5 minutes or until fragrant. Add the crushed tomatoes with liquid and puree, and bring to a simmer. Stir in the basil and oregano and season with the salt and pepper. Continue to simmer on reduced heat for 15 minutes. Adjust the consistency with water and season to taste.

KEVIN CRAWLEY

When Kevin Crawley traded in the kitchen for the classroom, it marked a return to familiar ground. The 1981 graduate of Johnson & Wales University in Providence, Rhode Island, returned to the culinary school to teach international cuisine, New World cuisine, and traditional European cuisine—all disciplines he's well familiar with after helming a French restaurant in Massachusetts for nearly 8 years. A runner for 2 decades, the two-time Boston Marathoner had for several years acted as race director for a 10-K fund-raiser, once running in his chef's coat. Besides teaching his students cooking skills, Crawley acts as faculty adviser to the boxing club, which helps develop the endurance you need for the food business. "I make them hit the hills in Providence," Crawley says. For more, go to jwu.edu.

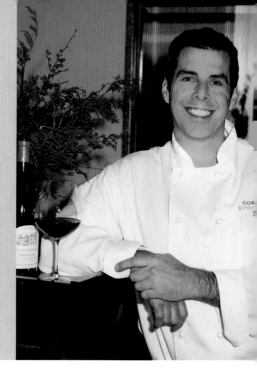

Chicken Stewed with Red Wine and Wild Mushrooms

`RECOVERY`

"This French-inspired dish is serious comfort food," Kevin Crawley says. "It's one-stop shopping for protein and carbs." Compared with many cuts of beef, chicken contains lower amounts of artery-clogging saturated fat and higher amounts of heart-healthy monounsaturated fat. Chicken is also a good source of niacin and B_6, two B vitamins that help your muscles use fat and carbohydrates for energy.

Makes 4 servings

PREP TIME: 15 MINUTES + REFRIGERATING THE PREPARED CHICKEN OVERNIGHT AND BRINGING CHICKEN TO ROOM TEMPERATURE FOR 1 HOUR / COOK TIME: 1 HOUR 30 MINUTES

2 tablespoons sugar

⅛ teaspoon ground ginger

⅛ teaspoon ground cinnamon

⅛ teaspoon ground coriander

⅛ teaspoon salt

⅛ teaspoon black pepper

Pinch of ground cloves

Pinch of ground nutmeg

(continued)

8 skinless chicken thighs

2 tablespoons extra virgin olive oil

1 small onion, diced

1 leek (white part only), diced

2 cloves garlic, minced

2 cups wild mushrooms, sliced

2 cups red wine

2 tablespoons tomato paste

1 cup canned diced tomatoes

2 bay leaves

1½ cups chicken stock

¼ cup chopped fresh parsley

Barley "Risotto" (recipe on opposite page)

Mix the sugar, ginger, cinnamon, coriander, salt, pepper, cloves, and nutmeg together. Rub the chicken with this mixture. Refrigerate the chicken overnight.

Remove the chicken from the fridge 1 hour before cooking. Heat the oil in a large stockpot over medium heat for 3 minutes. Brown the chicken on both sides and remove it from the pot; set aside. Add the onion, leek, garlic, and mushrooms. Cook, stirring frequently, over medium heat until the onion is golden, about 5 minutes. Add the wine, tomato paste, diced tomatoes, and bay leaves. Simmer until the mixture is reduced by one-quarter. Add the stock, then return the chicken to the pan and bring to a boil. Reduce the heat to low and simmer, covered, for 1 hour. Remove the chicken from the pot again. Skim the excess fat off the top. Simmer until the liquid thickens into a sauce (about 15 minutes). Stir in half the parsley. Place the chicken on plates, spoon the sauce on top, and garnish with parsley. Serve with Barley "Risotto" (recipe follows).

PER SERVING: 440 CALORIES • 32 G PROTEIN • 23 G CARBOHYDRATES • 14 G FAT

Barley "Risotto"

Kevin Crawley prepares this grain risotto-style. He adds stock little by little as the grain simmers, giving the dish a creamy texture. Pearl barley is an excellent source of fiber. One cup provides 6 grams, or nearly a quarter of the Daily Value. It also provides iron to help fight fatigue, selenium to protect immunity, and copper, which is important for joint flexibility.

Makes 4 servings

PREP TIME: 10 MINUTES / COOK TIME: 35 MINUTES

1 tablespoon extra virgin olive oil

½ small carrot, finely diced

½ rib celery, finely diced

½ small onion, finely diced

1¼ cups pearl barley

½ teaspoon chopped fresh thyme

½ teaspoon chopped fresh sage

½ teaspoon chopped fresh rosemary

½ tablespoon chopped fresh chives

4–5 cups vegetable or chicken stock

¼ cup grated Parmesan cheese

½ tablespoon unsalted butter (optional)

Snipped chives to taste

Heat the olive oil in a large saucepan. Add the carrot, celery, and onion. Sauté over medium heat for 2 to 3 minutes, stirring constantly. Add the barley and stir to coat the kernels with the oil. Stir in the herbs. Add enough stock to cover the barley and stir with a wooden spoon until the stock is absorbed into the barley, about 3 to 5 minutes.

Continue to add stock while stirring constantly until the barley is tender and has a creamy consistency (amount of stock varies depending on the type of barley). Stir in the cheese and butter, if desired. Garnish with snipped chives. Serve immediately.

PER SERVING: 350 CALORIES, 14 G PROTEIN, 55 G CARBOHYDRATES, 9 G FAT

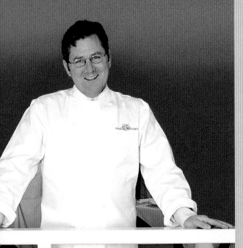

CHARLIE TROTTER

Before he was a chef, Charlie Trotter was a runner. As a college junior, Trotter decided to try the Chicago Marathon. He trained for only 4 weeks, but his athletic background—he was a trampolinist on his high-school gymnastics team—carried him to a 3:32 finish. Now the proprietor of an eponymous restaurant in Chicago, his hometown, Trotter has run more than a dozen additional marathons. His favorite, by far, is the Marathon du Médoc in Bordeaux, France, a vineyard tour that celebrates the region's grape harvest. "The race is Mardi Gras-esque," he says. "Half the runners are wearing costumes, there's a band every kilometer, and they serve wine on the course." For more, go to charlietrotters.com.

Chicken with Quinoa Tabbouleh   `RECOVERY`

Quinoa is a whole grain rich in carbohydrates and is as easily prepared as rice. One cup of raw quinoa is equivalent to about 3 cups cooked.

Makes 4 servings
PREP TIME: 15 MINUTES

Chicken

4 boneless, skinless chicken breast halves,
　　grilled and thinly sliced

Quinoa Tabbouleh

3 cups cooked quinoa, at room temperature

$\frac{1}{2}$ cup diced cucumber, skin on

$\frac{1}{4}$ cup diced red bell pepper

2 tablespoons chopped fresh flat-leaf
　　parsley

2 teaspoons chopped fresh mint

2 tablespoons extra virgin olive oil

1 tablespoon freshly squeezed lemon juice

2 tablespoons minced red onion

$1\frac{1}{2}$ tablespoons sherry vinegar

$\frac{1}{2}$ teaspoon kosher salt

$\frac{1}{8}$ teaspoon freshly ground black pepper

Parsley Vinaigrette

2 tablespoons freshly squeezed lemon juice

1½ tablespoons water

1 tablespoon olive oil

2½ tablespoons finely chopped flat-leaf parsley

Kosher salt and freshly ground black pepper

Tabbouleh

Combine the cooked quinoa, cucumber, bell pepper, parsley, mint, olive oil, lemon juice, red onion, and vinegar in a large bowl. Toss to mix. Season with salt and pepper.

Vinaigrette

Whisk together the lemon juice and water. Whisk in the olive oil, and then stir in the parsley. Season with salt and pepper.

Divide the cooked quinoa among 4 dishes or containers and top with the chicken. Drizzle with the vinaigrette.

PER SERVING: 410 CALORIES • 33 G PROTEIN • 32 G CARBOHYDRATES • 16 G FAT

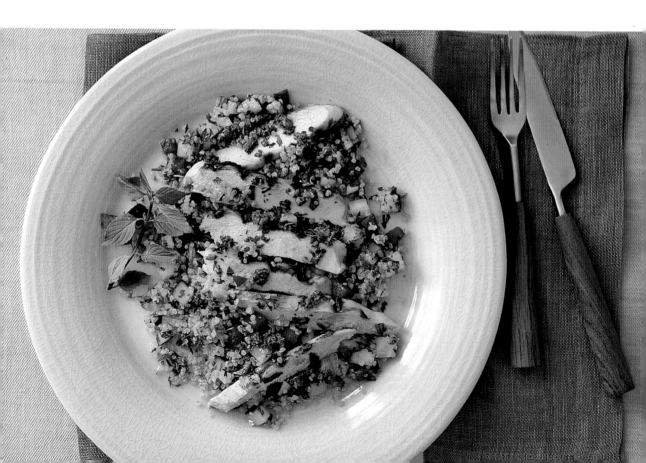

Orange-Cumin Glazed Pork Tenderloin

The leanest cut of pork, the tenderloin is a great source of protein and the nutrients thiamine and vitamin B$_6$, both critical for metabolizing carbohydrates, protein, and fat. It also provides bone-strengthening phosphorus, niacin, riboflavin, and zinc. A good source of iron, cumin aids digestion and may help prevent cancer. For more from Ivy Stark, see pages 6 and 76.

Makes 4 servings

PREP TIME: 15 MINUTES / COOK TIME: 1 HOUR, INCLUDING REST TIME

½ cup fresh orange juice

1–2 canned chipotles in adobo sauce

Peel from 1 orange (about 1 tablespoon)

1 tablespoon cumin seeds, lightly toasted

¼ teaspoon salt

2 pork tenderloins (1½ pounds each)

2 oranges, segmented (about 2 cups)

1 small red onion, thinly sliced

½ bunch cilantro, chopped (about ½–¾ cup)

Salt, to taste

Preheat the oven to 400°F.

Combine the orange juice, chipotles, orange peel, cumin seeds, and salt in a blender. Puree until smooth.

Place the pork tenderloins in a shallow dish and pour the orange mixture over them. Cover with plastic wrap and marinate the tenderloins in the refrigerator for at least 1 hour to overnight.

Take the tenderloins out of the marinade. Reserve the marinade.

Put the reserved marinade in a small saucepan and cook over medium heat until the sauce is reduced by half, about 10 to 12 minutes. Keep it warm.

Place the meat in shallow baking dish. Brush it with a little of the reserved marinade after 15 minutes. Bake for a total of 20 to 25 minutes, or until an instant-read thermometer registers 160°F when tested in center of the meat.

Remove the meat from the oven and let it rest in a warm place for 10 minutes; this seals in the juices before slicing.

Toss the orange segments, red onion, and cilantro in a small bowl with a little salt.

Cut the pork into ½"-thick slices before serving. Place the slices on a warm serving platter and drizzle them with the hot, reduced marinade. Surround the meat with the orange and red onion mixture.

PER SERVING: 313 CALORIES • 49 G PROTEIN • 15 G CARBOHYDRATES • 6 G FAT

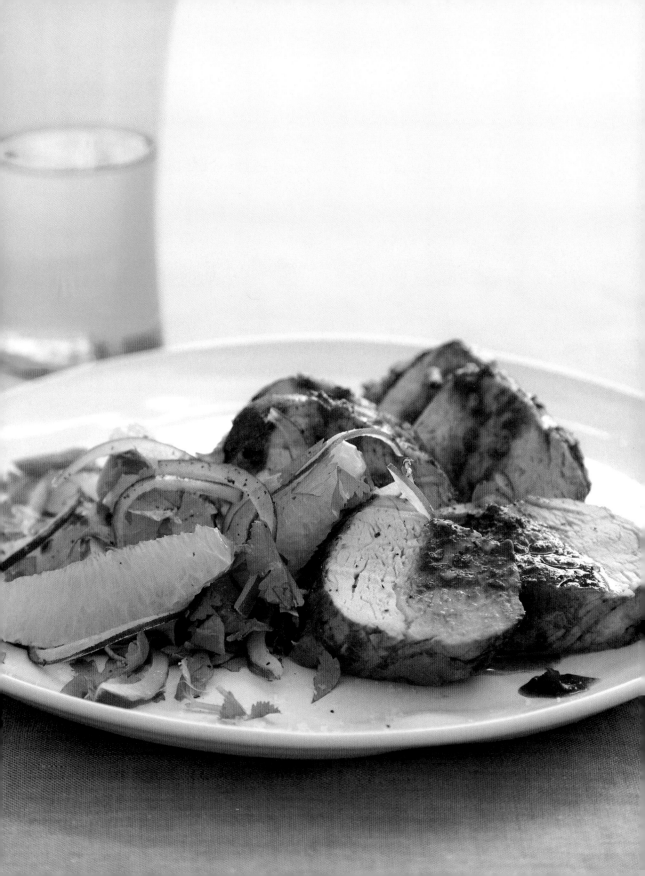

Pancetta-Wrapped Chicken Breast RECOVERY with Pesto Orzo and Grilled Zucchini

Chicken is an excellent source of protein. One 5-ounce chicken breast contains 35 grams, or 65 percent of the Daily Value. Chicken also provides energizing B vitamins, immunity-boosting selenium, iron, and zinc. A Greek pasta, orzo is shaped like rice and cooks quickly. An excellent source of vitamin C, zucchini also contains fiber, vitamin A, calcium, and iron—at only 20 calories a cup. For more from Matt Connors, see pages 38, 132, and 136.

Makes 4 servings

PREP TIME: 25 MINUTES / COOK TIME: 45 MINUTES

Pesto

1 cup fresh basil leaves, blanched	1 clove garlic, minced
2 tablespoons toasted pine nuts	2 tablespoons cold water
¼ cup grated Parmesan	1 teaspoon salt
¼ cup extra virgin olive oil	

Chicken

4 boneless, skinless chicken breasts	8 sprigs fresh thyme leaves
1 teaspoon salt	16 thin slices pancetta (about 6 ounces)
1 teaspoon pepper	Extra virgin olive oil for greasing the pan

Orzo

1 cup orzo	1 medium zucchini, sliced into ½" rounds
1 tomato, chopped	1–2 tablespoons extra virgin olive oil

Pesto

Place the basil, pine nuts, Parmesan, olive oil, garlic, water, and salt in a blender and pulse until smooth.

Chicken

Preheat oven to 400°F. Season the chicken with the salt, pepper, and thyme. Lay the slices of pancetta overlapping each other on a sheet of plastic wrap. Place the chicken on top at one end and roll it up in the pancetta, like a burrito. Remove the plastic and place the roll in a lightly oiled pan. Cook for 20 to 30 minutes, or until a thermometer inserted in the thickest portion registers 160°F and the juices run clear. Flip the roll halfway through the cooking time. Remove from the oven and slice.

Orzo

Cook the orzo according to package directions. Dress the zucchini slices with olive oil and grill over a medium-high grill until done, about 10 minutes, flipping halfway through. Toss the hot orzo with 2 tablespoons of pesto and chopped tomato. Serve with the sliced chicken breast and the grilled zucchini.

PER SERVING: 470 CALORIES, 41 G PROTEIN, 32 G CARBOHYDRATES, 20G FAT

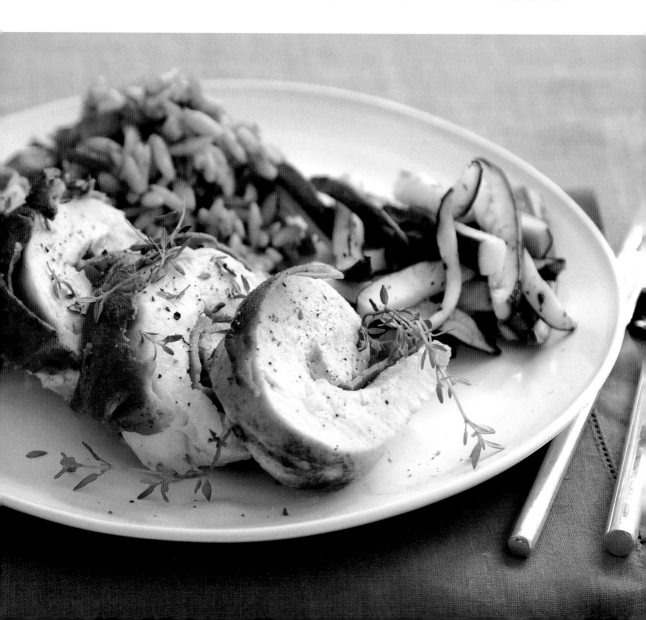

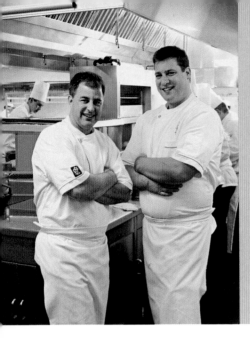

JONATHAN KRINN
AND JON MATHIESON

If a little competition is good for the workplace and for workouts, then Jonathan Krinn and Jon Mathieson are a case study for both. The two chefs behind Inox Restaurant in McLean, Virginia, together took up running and found their culinary partnership worked just as well on the road. "There's a lot of ripping on each other in the kitchen," says Krinn. "On a run, it's the same thing. Someone working with you pushes you harder than you'd ever push yourself." They lost a combined 100 pounds in a year and together finished in 2:36 at the 2007 National Half-Marathon in DC. For more, go to inoxrestaurant.com.

Roast Chicken with Pasta Gratin   `RECOVERY`

This gratin is hearty but healthy. "It's stick-to-your-ribs comfort food," says Jonathan Krinn. "The dish replenishes protein and carbs, perfect for after a run," Jon Mathieson says. Chicken provides B vitamins that help the muscles convert carbohydrates and fat into energy as well as immunity-enhancing selenium, fatigue-fighting iron, and zinc, which boosts recovery after injury.

Makes 4 servings
PREP TIME: 10 MINUTES / COOK TIME: 25 MINUTES

4 boneless, skinless chicken breasts

Salt and pepper to taste

1 onion, diced

2 carrots, cut into ½" dice

2 parsnips, ½" dice

1 celery root, ½" dice

Preheat the oven to 400°F. Season the chicken breasts with the salt and pepper. Sear 1 side for 5 minutes over medium-high heat in a nonstick, oven-proof, sauté or grill pan. Turn the chicken over and add the onion, carrots, parsnips, and celery root. As the vegetables begin to brown (about 6 minutes), turn them over and place the pan in the oven until the chicken is cooked

(7 to 10 minutes). Remove the chicken and let it rest while the vegetables finish cooking in the oven (about 5 minutes more). Serve with Pasta Gratin (recipe below).

PER SERVING: 210 CALORIES • 28 G PROTEIN • 15 G CARBOHYDRATES • 4 G FAT

Pasta Gratin

Makes 4 servings

PREP TIME: 10 MINUTES / COOK TIME: 5–8 MINUTES

12 ounces farfalle noodles

2 tablespoons part-skim ricotta

1 tablespoon mascarpone (or 2 tablespoons cream cheese total)

1 tablespoon low-fat cream cheese

1 ounce goat cheese

2 tablespoons half-and-half (optional)

3 tablespoons grated Parmesan cheese

Salt and pepper to taste

Follow the package directions to cook the pasta al dente. Mix together the ricotta, mascarpone, cream cheese, and goat cheese; thin with half-and-half if desired. Toss the cooked pasta with the cheese mixture, pour it into a 2-quart casserole dish, and top with the Parmesan. Place it under the broiler (450°F) until the cheese has browned, about 5 to 8 minutes.

PER SERVING: 410 CALORIES • 16 G PROTEIN • 65 G CARBOHYDRATES • 8 G FAT

Kota Kapama (Cinnamon Chicken)

"This version of a Greek dish is low in saturated fat because I use olive oil instead of butter or cream," says Cat Cora. But because it is stewed for an hour, the chicken is bursting with flavor. Serve over a bed of cooked quinoa or another favorite grain. For more from Cat Cora, see pages 20, 145, 155, 157, and 174.

Makes 4 servings

PREP TIME: 20 MINUTES / COOK TIME: 1 HOUR 10 MINUTES

1 whole chicken (2½–3 pounds), cut into 8 pieces

1 teaspoon ground cinnamon

2 teaspoons kosher salt

1 teaspoon freshly ground black pepper

1½ tablespoons extra virgin olive oil

2 coarsely chopped medium yellow onions

3 garlic cloves + 2 garlic cloves, minced

½ cup dry white wine

1 cup chicken stock

1 can (16 ounces) tomato paste

1 tablespoon chopped fresh oregano

Rinse the chicken and pat it dry with paper towels. Mix the cinnamon, kosher salt, and pepper in a small bowl. Rub the spice mix all over the chicken pieces.

Heat the olive oil in a large, deep skillet over high heat (a 12″ skillet with sides about 2½″ to 3″ high will allow you to brown all the chicken at once). Add the chicken to the oil and brown for about 4 to 5 minutes on each side, until the pieces are well browned all over. Remove the chicken and set aside.

Lower the heat to medium-high and add the onions and three-fifths of the minced garlic cloves. Cook for about 3 minutes, stirring constantly, until the onions have softened and are a rich golden-brown. Add the wine. When the wine has evaporated, add the water, chicken stock, tomato paste, oregano, and remaining 2 garlic cloves. Return the chicken to the pan. The liquid should cover about three-quarters of the chicken pieces. Cover the pot and simmer over low heat for about an hour or until the chicken is tender and thoroughly cooked. Season the finished sauce with kosher salt and pepper to taste.

PER SERVING (IF PREPARED WITHOUT THE SKIN):
360 CALORIES • 40 G PROTEIN • 18 G CARBOHYDRATES • 11 G FAT

PER SERVING (IF PREPARED WITH THE SKIN):
650 CALORIES • 47 G PROTEIN • 18 G CARBOHYDRATES • 41 G FAT

Stir-Fried Beef with Scallions and Mushrooms

A classic Chinese brown sauce acts as a flavorful gravy on simple stir-fries of beef, chicken, pork, tofu, or vegetables. A lean cut of beef, sirloin provides protein, iron, and calcium. Look for grass-fed beef, which is lower in overall fat and has a higher concentration of good fats such as omega-3 fatty acids, which benefit cardiovascular health, and cancer-fighting conjugated linoleic acids. For more from Grace Parisi, see page 94.

Makes 4 servings

PREP TIME: 20 MINUTES / COOK TIME: 15 MINUTES FOR THE STIR-FRY AND SAUCE

¼ cup peanut oil

¾ pound oyster mushrooms, stems trimmed

4 scallions, cut into 2" lengths

1 top sirloin (¾ pound), 1" thick, cut into ⅓"-thick x 4"-long slices

Salt and freshly ground black pepper, to taste

1 garlic clove, minced

Classic Chinese Brown Sauce (recipe page 122)

Prepare the Chinese Brown Sauce according to directions on page 122. Set aside.

Heat a wok or large skillet over high heat until very hot to the touch. Add 2 tablespoons of the oil and heat until shimmering. Add the oyster mushrooms and scallions and stir-fry until tender and browned in spots, about 5 minutes. Transfer the mixture to a plate.

Return the wok or skillet to high heat and add the remaining 2 tablespoons oil. Season the beef lightly with the salt and pepper. Add the beef to the pan in a single layer and cook, turning once until browned, about 2 minutes. Add the garlic and cook, tossing it with the meat, just until fragrant, about 30 seconds.

Return the mushrooms and scallions to the pan and stir until heated through. Add the sauce and cook, just until heated and bubbling, about 1 minute longer. Serve immediately over rice.

(continued)

Classic Chinese Brown Sauce

¾ cup low-sodium chicken broth

2 tablespoons light soy sauce

1 tablespoon Chinese cooking wine or dry sherry

1½ teaspoons cornstarch dissolved in 1 tablespoon water

Pinch of sugar

1 tablespoon prepared black bean garlic sauce (found in Asian markets)

2 scallions (white and tender green parts), chopped

1 tablespoon peeled and minced fresh ginger

1 tablespoon peanut oil

Combine the broth, soy sauce, cooking wine, cornstarch slurry, and sugar in a small measuring cup.

Combine the black bean garlic sauce with the scallions and ginger in another cup.

Heat the oil in a small saucepan or skillet over high heat until smoking. Add the black bean mixture and cook just until fragrant, about 1 minute. Stir the stock mixture, add it to the saucepan, and bring it to a boil. Reduce the heat to medium and simmer the sauce until thickened and glossy, 1 to 2 minutes longer.

PER SERVING: 335 CALORIES • 23 G PROTEIN • 11 G CARBOHYDRATES • 22 G FAT

Tiny Tacos

These tacos are made by filling Tostitos Baked! Scoops. Ten of these filled, bite-size tacos are only 210 total calories. For more from Devin Alexander, see pages 124 and 192.

Makes 1 serving

PREP TIME: 10 MINUTES / COOK TIME: 2–3 MINUTES

10 Tostitos Baked! Scoops

¼ cup finely shredded romaine

2 tablespoons finely chopped tomato

½ ounce (about 2½ tablespoons) finely shredded Cabot's 75% light Cheddar cheese, or any low-fat Cheddar

1 teaspoon lower-sodium taco seasoning

2 tablespoons water

2 ounces 96% lean ground beef

1 tablespoon mild or hot red taco sauce

Arrange the Scoops side by side on a plate.

Mix the lettuce, tomato, and cheese in a medium bowl until well combined. Divide evenly among the Scoops (about 1½ teaspoons per Scoop)

Add the taco seasoning to a small bowl and stir the water into the seasoning, continuing to stir until it has no lumps. Set aside.

Preheat a small, nonstick skillet over medium-high heat. Add the beef to the skillet and use a wooden spoon to coarsely crumble the meat as it cooks. When the beef is no longer pink, after about 1 to 2 minutes, stir in the seasoning mixture. When no liquid remains, after about 1 minute, remove the skillet from the heat. Divide the meat evenly among the Scoops atop the lettuce mixture (about 1 teaspoon in each). Dollop the top of each with taco sauce, and serve immediately.

PER SERVING: 210 CALORIES • 18 G PROTEIN • 19 G CARBOHYDRATES • 6 G FAT

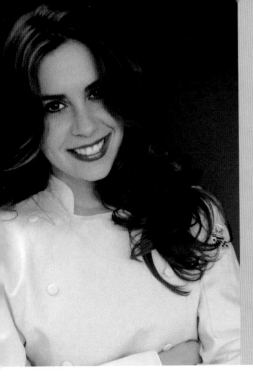

DEVIN ALEXANDER

As a teenager, Devin Alexander always struggled to maintain a healthy weight. "I was gaining 10 to 15 pounds a year, and I was constantly on a diet," says the chef, who is based in Los Angeles. She started experimenting with ways to create healthier versions of her favorite meals, such as using cooking spray instead of oil, and espresso powder to add richness to a lower-fat chocolate cake. Revamping her diet and running 3 miles nearly every day has helped Alexander maintain her 55-pound weight loss for 15 years, and she preaches what she practices on FitTV's *Healthy Decadence with Devin Alexander,* in cookbooks such as *The Most Decadent Diet Ever,* and in *The Biggest Loser* cookbooks based on the reality television show. For more, go to devinalexander.com.

Superstuffed Steak Soft Taco

QUICK AND EASY   RECOVERY

A lean cut of beef, reduced-fat cheese, and cooking spray reduce the calories and fat in this recipe. Lean meat can be prone to toughness from overcooking. "Always start cooking it on high heat," Devin Alexander says.

Makes 1 serving

PREP TIME: 15 MINUTES / COOK TIME: 7–9 MINUTES

4 ounces top round steak

1 low-carb flour tortilla (8" diameter)

½–1 teaspoon salt-free Mexican or
    Southwest seasoning

⅛ teaspoon garlic powder

Pinch of salt, or to taste

⅔ cup finely shredded romaine

¼ cup chopped tomato

1 ounce shredded Cabot's 75% light
    Cheddar cheese

1 tablespoon red taco sauce

2 tablespoons fresh cilantro

Preheat the oven to 400°F. Place the steak between 2 sheets of waxed paper. Use the toothed side of a meat mallet to pound both sides of the steak until it's ⅓" thick. Cut it into ¼" strips. Wrap the tortilla in foil and place it directly on the oven rack to warm for 5 minutes. Mix together the Mexican seasoning, garlic powder, and salt. Add the steak strips and toss to coat evenly. Preheat a nonstick skillet to medium-high. Mist it lightly with olive oil cooking spray. Add the steak strips in a single layer and cook 2 to 4 minutes. Place the tortilla on a plate and spoon the steak strips over half of it. Top it evenly with the lettuce, tomato, cheese, taco sauce, and cilantro. Fold in half.

PER SERVING: 320 CALORIES • 40 G PROTEIN • 17 G CARBOHYDRATES • 14 G FAT

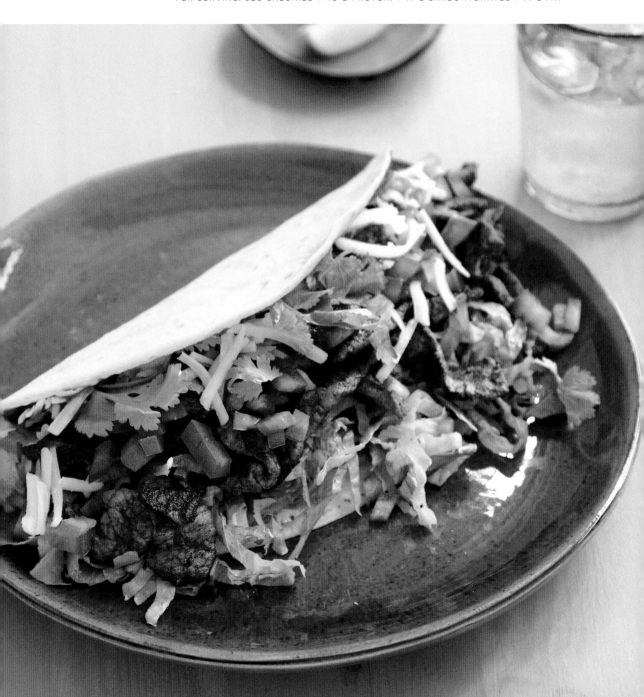

Acapulco-Style Mahi Mahi Ceviche   `RECOVERY`

This mahi mahi ceviche was inspired by dishes at Richard Sandoval's restaurant Madeiras, located in Acapulco. It uses red curry pasta (found at Asian groceries or gourmet markets) and chili sauce to spice up raw fish. For more from Richard Sandoval, see pages 66 and 169.

Makes 4 servings

PREP TIME: 10 MINUTES + 30 MINUTES REFRIGERATION TIME / COOK TIME: 7 MINUTES

3 ounces Malibu rum

1 tablespoon red Thai curry paste

¼ cup ketchup

2 tablespoons coconut milk (unsweetened)

2 tablespoons chili sauce

1 tablespoon extra virgin olive oil

1 tablespoon chopped fresh ginger

1 tablespoon chopped lemongrass

2 sushi-grade mahi mahi fillets (8 ounces each), skinned and cubed

1 tablespoon chopped cilantro

Mix together the rum, curry paste, ketchup, coconut milk, and chili sauce in a medium bowl. Set aside.

Heat the olive oil in a medium sauté pan over medium heat. Add the ginger and lemongrass and cook, stirring frequently, for 2 minutes or until fragrant. Add the curry paste mixture and simmer 5 minutes to blend the flavors and reduce the rum. Remove from heat and cool.

Mix the curry paste mixture, mahi mahi, and cilantro in a large bowl, making sure to coat fish evenly.

Set aside for 30 minutes in the refrigerator, allowing the flavors to meld. Serve in individual bowls or cocktail glasses.

PER SERVING: 220 CALORIES • 22 G PROTEIN • 13 G CARBOHYDRATES • 6 G FAT

Alaskan Salmon in a Barley, Spring Vegetables, and Port Reduction

Fatty cold-water fish like salmon contains heart-healthy omega-3 fatty acids and is a good source of protein. Wild-caught salmon has the most nutritional benefit. For more from Mark Monette, see pages 47 and 70.

Makes 4 servings

PREP TIME: 20 MINUTES + 20 MINUTES REFRIGERATION TIME / COOK TIME: 1 HOUR 15 MINUTES

4 Alaska salmon fillets (6 ounces each)

1 shallot, chopped

2 cloves garlic, chopped

3 tablespoons unsalted butter

½ cup diced onion

½ cup diced celery root

½ cup diced carrot

2 bay leaves

6 black peppercorns

2 sprigs thyme

¾ cup barley or pearled barley

4 cups duck, chicken, or vegetarian stock

12 sprigs watercress

¼ cup fresh English peas

6 fresh basil leaves, chopped

Port Reduction

2 cups port

2 tablespoons sherry vinegar

2 tablespoons sweet soy sauce or balsamic vinegar

Salt and pepper to taste

¼ cup extra virgin olive oil

(continued)

Sauté the shallots and garlic in butter in a medium sauté pan. Add the onion, celery root, and carrot, and continue to cook, stirring frequently, for 5 minutes or until celery root and carrot are tender. Make a bouquet garni by wrapping a small square of cheesecloth or a coffee filter around 2 bay leaves, 6 black peppercorns, and 2 sprigs of thyme, and secure it at the top with clean twine or string. Add the barley, stock, and bouquet garni and let it simmer for 45 minutes, or until the grains are tender. Make a bouquet garni by wrapping a small square of cheesecloth or a coffee filter around 2 bay leaves, 6 black peppercorns, and 2 sprigs of thyme, and secure it at the top with clean twine or string.

Strain the barley and remove the bouquet garni when barley is cooked. Let stand.

To make the port reduction, place the port, vinegar, soy sauce, salt, and pepperin a saucepot and reduce over medium simmer to a syrup consistency, about 20 to 30 minutes or longer. Chill for 20 minutes and blend in the olive oil.

Sear salmon in a sauté pan over medium-high heat on both sides until medium-rare, 2 to 4 minutes, depending on the fillet thickness.

Toss the watercress and peas into the barley. Mix in $\frac{1}{2}$ cup of the port reduction. Divide the barley mixture among 4 plates, place a salmon fillet on top of each plate, sprinkle with the chopped basil, and serve.

PER SERVING: 630 CALORIES • 45 G PROTEIN • 47 G CARBOHYDRATES • 26 G FAT

LEWIS BUTLER

Lewis Butler began running about 15 years ago in his native Montreal to "get fit and get some sun," he says. Now a resident of the sunny beach town of Laguna Beach, California, where he oversees the restaurant Splashes at the Surf & Sand Resort, Butler competes in up to four half-marathons a year (with a PR of 1:27). "In a 5-K you feel like you must run it as fast as you can. To run a marathon you really need to spend time training," he says. "That's why the half is the perfect challenge." For more, go to surfandsandresort.com.

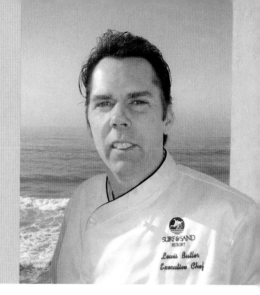

Baked Asian-Style Salmon

TRAINING

Lewis Butler likes to enjoy this salmon dish the night before a race for its protein, carbohydrates, and healthy fats. "It is originally a French recipe, but at home I blend it with Asian flavors," he says. Baking the fish and vegetables in parchment paper means no oil is needed for cooking and nutrients are better retained. The dish can be prepared in advance and refrigerated before cooking. It also works on the grill, with foil substituting for the parchment paper. Along with benefiting cardiovascular health, the omega-3 fatty acids in salmon help fight joint pain by reducing inflammation.

Makes 6 servings

PREP TIME: 25 MINUTES / COOK TIME: 40–45 MINUTES

2 tablespoons butter

4 medium onions, thinly sliced

½ carrot, sliced into ribbons with a peeler

2 baby bok choy heads, chopped

1 green or red bell pepper, diced

2 cups bean sprouts

2 limes

⅓ cup soy sauce

⅓ cup teriyaki sauce

6 salmon fillets (5 ounces each, about 2 pounds total)

10 mint leaves

(continued)

Preheat the oven to 375°F. Melt the butter over low heat in a small skillet. Add the onions. Cook 25 minutes, or until caramelized. Mix the carrot, bok choy, bell pepper, bean sprouts, and caramelized onions in a bowl. Grate the limes' peel. Mix the grated peel, soy sauce, and teriyaki sauce in another bowl. Coat the salmon with the sauce mixture. Cut the rind off the limes and slice them. Tear 6 pieces of 12″ × 12″ parchment paper or foil. Divide the vegetables into 6 portions and place a portion on each piece of paper, 2″ from the bottom. Top each with 1 piece of salmon, 1 or 2 mint leaves, a drizzle of sauce, and a lime slice. Fold the top of each piece of paper over the salmon. Starting in an upper corner, fold and crease the paper edges all the way around to seal the packet. It will resemble a half circle. Bake the packets on a sheet for 15 to 20 minutes, remove from the oven, and serve in the paper.

PER SERVING: 330 CALORIES • 35 G PROTEIN • 18 G CARBOHYDRATES • 14 G FAT

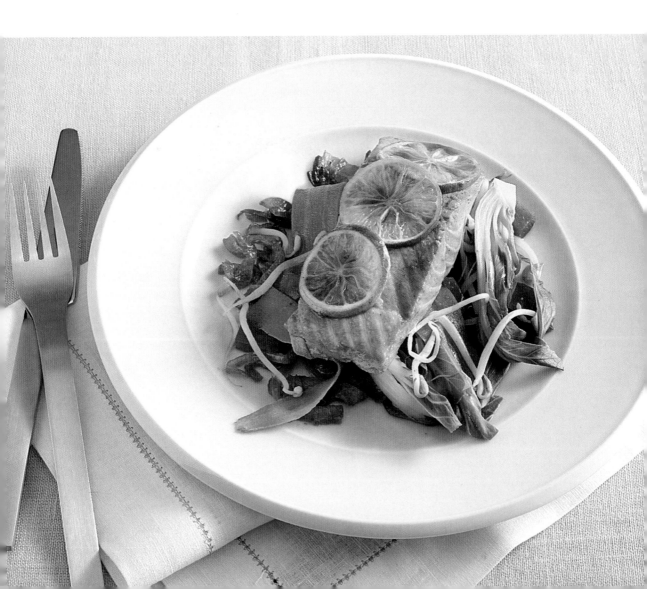

RICH VELLANTE

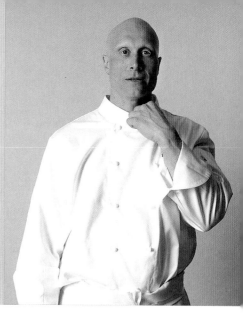

Each year since 2002, Rich Vellante has competed in the Boston Marathon, his hometown race, to raise money for Boston's Dana-Farber Cancer Institute. With a PR of 3:59, the executive chef of Legal Sea Foods restaurants fuels up with seafood, as do many of his fellow marathoners. But his day job might give him a leg up on the competition. "The pressure of training for a marathon and of working in a restaurant helps keep you focused," he says. "There are plenty of opportunities to panic in a restaurant or during a run, but you have to stay calm and work through them." For more, go to legalseafoods.com.

Cape Cod Baked Scallops with Lime   `TRAINING`

Seafood is a great source of high-quality protein and heart-healthy omega-3 fatty acids. Vellante developed this recipe during a vacation on Cape Cod.

Makes 4 servings

PREP TIME: 15 MINUTES / COOK TIME: 20–25 MINUTES

2 pounds sea scallops (fresh or thawed from frozen)

¼ cup chopped fresh basil

1 teaspoon grated lime or lemon peel

½ teaspoon cumin

1 tablespoon extra virgin olive oil

1 tablespoon freshly squeezed lime juice

1½ teaspoons kosher salt

Black pepper, to taste

½ cup white wine

¾–1 cup Italian bread crumbs

2 tablespoons olive oil

Preheat the oven to 400°F. Rinse the scallops and pat them dry. Remove and discard each "foot" (the little tough piece on the side of each scallop). Put the scallops in a glass or ceramic bowl and toss with the basil, lime or lemon peel, cumin, olive oil, lime juice, salt, and pepper.

Place the scallops in a baking dish.

Sprinkle the wine over the top of the scallops. Lightly cover the scallops with the bread crumbs. Drizzle the olive oil over the top. Bake for 20 to 25 minutes, until the scallops are cooked through and the tops are nicely browned.

PER SERVING: 400 CALORIES • 40 G PROTEIN • 21 G CARBOHYDRATES • 13 G FAT

Grilled Salmon with Vegetable Couscous and Artichoke Vinaigrette

Protein-packed salmon, like other oily cold-water fish, is a great source of omega-3 fatty acids, which benefit the heart and reduce the inflammation associated with joint pain. For more from Matt Connors, see pages 38, 116, and 136.

Makes 4 servings

PREP TIME: 20 MINUTES / COOK TIME: 15–25 MINUTES

Vinaigrette:

6 baby artichokes, cooked, or substitute
with artichokes jarred in olive oil

1/4 cup white wine vinegar

1 shallot, sliced

1 teaspoon Dijon mustard

3/4 cup extra virgin olive oil

1 teaspoon chopped fresh tarragon

Place the artichokes, vinegar, shallot, mustard, olive oil, and tarragon in a blender and blend until emulsified. Warm over a low flame in a pot.

Couscous:

1/2 medium tomato, diced

1/4 cup chopped and cooked fresh asparagus

1/4 cup fresh peas, blanched

1/4 cup chopped and cooked green beans

1/2 cup cooked couscous

2 tablespoons extra virgin olive oil

2 tablespoons fresh lemon juice

2 tablespoons sliced basil

2 tablespoons diced fresh chives

Toss the tomato, asparagus, peas, green beans, couscous, oil, lemon juice, basil, and chives well. Set aside.

Fish:

4 salmon fillets (6 ounces each), skin removed

Season the salmon with salt and pepper and sear on a grill pan for 2 minutes on each side, or until the fish is opaque.

Divide the couscous mixture among 4 plates and drizzle with the warm vinaigrette (about 2 tablespoons per fillet. You will have leftover vinaigrette). Serve.

PER SERVING: 590 CALORIES • 39 G PROTEIN • 23 G CARBOHYDRATES • 38 G FAT

ANDREW DORNENBURG AND KAREN PAGE

Andrew Dornenburg and Karen Page have run six marathons and 11 half-marathons between them. "For our honeymoon in 1990, we ate our way through Quebec City and Montreal, and ran the Montreal International Marathon on our last day in Canada," says Dornenburg, who set a PR of 3:23:13 in Chicago in 2002. Having written seven books about food and chefs, the authors say they run to eat, and have even lost weight while on deadline. "A few years ago, we each lost 10-plus pounds while researching and writing *What to Drink with What You Eat*," Page says, "which proves that peak flavor combinations are so satisfying that quality outstrips any need for quantity." For more, go to becomingachef.com.

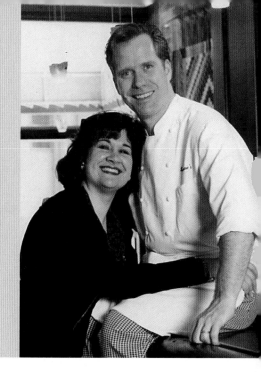

Grilled Tuna with Plum Salsa and Boiled New Potatoes

RECOVERY

"This is one of my favorite dishes," Karen Page says. Plums help the body better absorb iron and are rich in the immunity-boosting antioxidant vitamin C. If ripe plums aren't available, enhance the flavor by poaching underripe ones in chicken stock and adding honey. You can make the salsa up to 2 hours in advance. For more from Andrew Dornenburg and Karen Page, see page 46.

Makes 4 servings

PREP TIME: 20 MINUTES / COOK TIME: 15 MINUTES

4 ripe plums, halved and pits removed

1 red onion, thinly sliced

1 clove garlic, minced

2 sprigs fresh thyme, lightly chopped

1 tablespoon Champagne vinegar or balsamic vinegar

3 tablespoons extra virgin olive oil + additional for rubbing

1 teaspoon honey

8 organic new potatoes (about 3 pounds)

Kosher salt

1 tablespoon chopped chives

4 sushi-grade tuna steaks (about 6 ounces and 1" thick each)

Sea salt and freshly ground pepper

(continued on page 135)

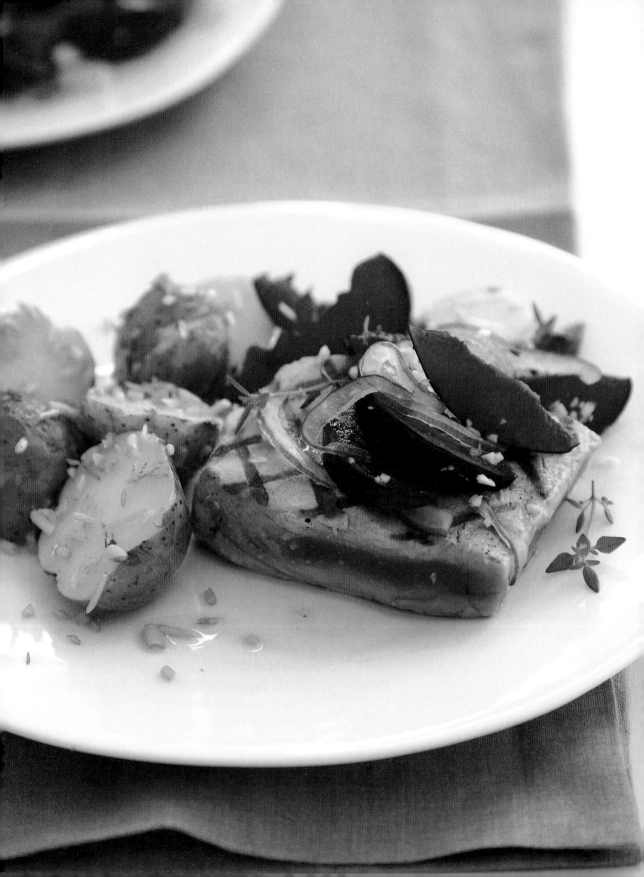

Salsa

Cut the plum halves into thin (⅛″) slices. Reserve any juice. Combine the plum slices, onion, and garlic in a bowl. Add the thyme, vinegar, olive oil, reserved plum juice, and honey. Stir together and set aside.

Potatoes

Boil the potatoes for 10–12 minutes or until they are soft enough that a fork can go through them. Season them with a sprinkle of kosher salt and chopped chives.

Tuna

Coat a grill rack or stovetop ridged skillet with cooking spray. Preheat the grill or the pan. Take the tuna out of the refrigerator and let it warm up for a few minutes.

Rub the tuna steaks with a little olive oil, sea salt, and freshly ground black pepper.

Coat the grill rack with cooking spray and preheat the grill. Cook the tuna steaks for about 2 minutes on each side, or until the fish is just opaque (for rare tuna). Place the tuna on individual plates or on a large platter, and top with the salsa. Serve with the potatoes.

PER SERVING: 390 CALORIES • 46 G PROTEIN • 35 G CARBOHYDRATES • 6 G FAT

Pan-Roasted Halibut with Chickpeas and Roasted Tomato Pasta

Halibut is a lean, low-calorie source of protein. Chickpeas, also known as garbanzo beans, contain fiber, which helps lower cholesterol levels. They are also a good source for folate and magnesium, both of which are good for your heart and cardiovascular system. Cooked tomatoes provide the cancer-fighting antioxidant lycopene. For more recipes by Matt Connors, see pages 38, 116, and 132.

Makes 4 servings

PREP TIME: 10 MINUTES / COOK TIME: 15 MINUTES

Halibut

4 halibut fillets (6 ounces each)

Salt and freshly ground black pepper to taste

2 tablespoons extra virgin olive oil

Season the fillets with salt and pepper. Heat the oil in a large sauté pan and sear the fillets for 2 minutes on each side , or until the fish flakes easily and it's crisp and golden. Place in a warm oven until ready to serve.

Pasta e fagioli

½ cup ditali pasta

1½ tablespoons extra virgin olive oil

2 teaspoons minced fresh garlic

½ cup high-quality canned tomatoes, preferably packed in oil

1 cup chicken stock

½ cup canned chickpeas (garbanzo beans), drained and rinsed

4 thick slices soppressata (Italian dry-cured salami), diced (about 5 ounces)

½ cup diced zucchini

20 fresh basil leaves (about ½ cup loosely packed), sliced

6 tablespoons freshly grated Parmesan cheese

Cook the pasta according to package directions. Drain. Heat the olive oil in a large sauté pan over medium heat and sauté the garlic until golden. Add the tomatoes, chicken stock, chickpeas, soppressata, zucchini, and basil, and simmer for 5 minutes over medium-low heat, stirring occasionally. Toss with the Parmesan, and divide the pasta e fagioli among 4 shallow bowls. Top each bowl with a halibut fillet and serve.

PER SERVING: 540 CALORIES • 53 G PROTEIN • 19 G CARBOHYDRATES • 27 G FAT

MARIA HINES

Maria Hines loves running in Seattle, for the weather—she doesn't mind the rain—and the views. "On an 8-mile trail run through the woods of Mount Si, you gain more than 3,000 feet," says the San Diego native. "The higher you get, the more beautiful the view of Snoqualmie Valley. You can hear yourself think." A yoga practitioner, Hines also rock-climbs, and has set her sights on scaling El Capitán in Yosemite National Park. As the chef-owner of Tilth, only the second U.S. restaurant to be certified organic by the rigorous standards of Oregon Tilth, she is focused on local, sustainable food, such as Penn Cove mussels and Walla Walla onions. But she is the first to admit her eating habits aren't always race-ready. "I drink coffee, beer, and bourbon, and eat doughnuts," she says. "But not all at once!" For more, go to tilthrestaurant.com.

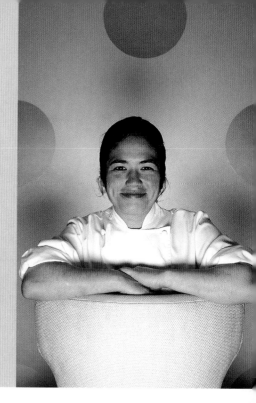

Poached Albacore Tuna with Pappardelle

Albacore tuna is a good source of protein, vitamins A and B$_{12}$, niacin, and selenium. It also provides omega-3 fatty acids, which can help lower levels of low-density lipoprotein (LDL or so-called "bad") cholesterol and reduce the risk of heart disease. If you're concerned about seafood sustainability, Pacific stocks of albacore are at record or near-record highs. For more from Maria Hines, see page 74.

Makes 4 servings

PREP TIME: 15 MINUTES / COOK TIME: 35–40 MINUTES

12 ounces pappardelle

4 tablespoons extra virgin olive oil

1 cup diced celery

1 cup diced onion

¼ cup coarsely chopped parsley

1 teaspoon minced garlic

¼ cup capers, drained

2 tablespoons minced preserved lemon, or use grated peel of 1 lemon

2 cups water

(continued)

2 cups good-quality white wine

1 bay leaf

3 sprigs thyme

Kosher salt and ground white pepper, to taste

4 Albacore tuna fillets (6 ounces each)

½ cup oven-dried tomatoes, or sun-dried tomatoes packed in oil

¼ cup freshly grated Parmigiano Reggiano

½ teaspoon coarsely chopped tarragon

½ teaspoon coarsely chopped chives

Cook the pappardelle according to package directions, and set aside. Separately, heat 2 tablespoons of the olive oil in a large skillet over medium heat. Add the celery, onion, and garlic and cook for 5 minutes or until soft. Add the capers, lemon, water, wine, bay leaf, thyme, kosher salt, and pepper, and let come to a simmer. Simmer for 10 minutes, then add the uncooked albacore tuna and simmer for 6 minutes (or longer if needed). Take the tuna out of the bouillon and set aside.

Strain out all the boullion ingredients (throw out thyme sprigs and bay leaf) and reserve. Discard the liquid, bay leaf, and thyme. Heat the remaining 2 tablespoons of the olive oil in a large skillet over medium heat. Add the tomatoes, cooked pasta, and the reserved bouillon ingredients to the skillet and cook for 5 to 7 minutes. Toss with the cheese, tarragon, and chives and serve.

PER SERVING: 570 CALORIES • 54 G PROTEIN • 77 G CARBOHYDRATES • 5 G FAT

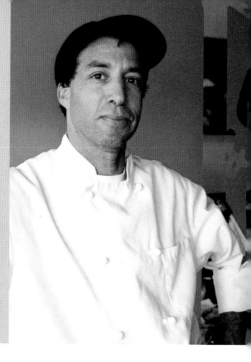

SARIG AGASI

Sarig Agasi qualified for Boston with a 3:01 he earned running his first-ever marathon in 2004 in New York City. His Boston time? 3:01. Agasi's enthusiasm for his new sport—he'd been running for only about a year—prompted him to create this Salmon and Edamame Penne and to put it on the menu of Zely & Ritz, the restaurant where he is chef and co-owner. The tapas restaurant in Raleigh, North Carolina, features the pasta as a special when local races are being held. "But if you come in and you're training and it's not listed," says the Israeli native, "please, just ask." It must be working for the chef. A year and a half after Boston, he broke 3 hours, finishing the 2006 Outer Banks Marathon in 2:55. For more, go to zelyandritz.com.

Salmon and Edamame Penne

TRAINING

Packed with protein, heart-disease-preventing omega-3 fatty acids, and plenty of whole grain carbs, this pasta reflects Sarig Agasi's background. It fuses classical French cooking techniques (in this case, the preparation of the salmon) with his Israeli childhood's Mediterranean flavors including olives and capers.

Makes 2 servings

PREP TIME: 15 MINUTES / COOK TIME: 30 MINUTES

- 3 teaspoons extra virgin olive oil
- ¼ cup diced red onion
- ¼ cup diced green bell pepper
- ⅛ cup (about 10) diced green Manzanillo olives
- ⅛ cup capers
- 1 tablespoon chopped fresh sage

- 1 tablespoon chopped fresh oregano
- ¼ cup diced yellow onion
- 2 medium tomatoes, diced
- 6 ounces whole wheat penne pasta
- ½ cup shelled edamame
- 2 (5-ounce) wild salmon fillets, with skin

Heat 1 teaspoon of the olive oil in a large skillet over medium heat. Add the red onion and bell pepper and cook, stirring frequently, for 3 minutes or until pepper is tender. Stir in the olives, capers, sage, and oregano. Remove from the heat. Heat 1 teaspoon of the olive oil in a pot over medium heat, add the yellow onion and cook, stirring frequently, until golden-brown. Add the tomatoes. Cover and cook over low heat for 10 minutes. Remove the pot from the heat and use a

(continued)

hand blender to mix the tomatoes in the pot. Stir the olive mixture into the tomato mixture and set aside. Boil the pasta according to the package directions, adding the edamame about 2 minutes before the pasta is ready. Drain. Heat the remaining teaspoon of olive oil in a nonstick sauté pan over high heat and cook the salmon, skin side down, for 1 minute. Lower the heat to medium and cook for another 5 minutes. Flip and cook for another minute. Mix the pasta in a bowl with three-quarters of the tomato sauce and divide between 2 plates or large shallow bowls. Top the pasta with the salmon and distribute the remaining sauce across the salmon.

PER SERVING: 710 CALORIES • 46 G PROTEIN • 77 G CARBOHYDRATES • 25 G FAT

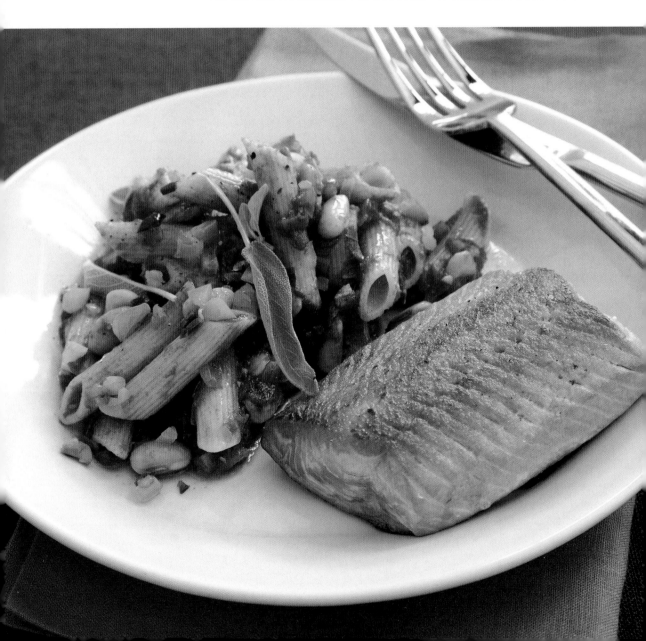

Salmon Baked in Paper

Salmon is high in protein and a good source of omega-3 fatty acids, which benefit the cardiovascular system. Edwyn Ferrari says, "Baking in parchment paper is very healthy and very easy." It helps retain nutrients while allowing flavors to better blend. For more from Edwyn Ferrari, see page 8.

Makes 2 servings

PREP TIME: 20 MINUTES / COOK TIME: 22 MINUTES

2 tablespoons low-sodium soy sauce

½ teaspoon toasted sesame oil

2 teaspoons fresh lemon or lime juice

1 teaspoon sugar

Pinch of sea salt

Pinch of black pepper

½ teaspoon roasted sesame seeds

2 scallions, cut into 2"pieces

3 baby carrots, halved

3 baby squash, halved, or 1 cup yellow and green squash, cut into rounds

1 tablespoon extra-virgin olive oil

1 (16-ounce) wild salmon fillet, skin removed

Combine the soy sauce, sesame oil, lemon juice, sugar, sea salt, pepper, and sesame seeds in a large bowl and set aside. Add the scallions, carrots, and squash, and toss to coat.

Lay a piece of 12″ × 16″ parchment paper flat and brush on the olive oil to cover. Place the salmon in the center of the parchment. Place the coated vegetables on top and around the sides of the salmon. Lift up and bring together the 2 long sides of the paper and fold it over to create a seal. Fold over the 2 shorter sides to create seals as well. Bake at 375°F for about 15 minutes for medium-rare to medium, or 22 minutes for medium to well done.

PER SERVING: 444 CALORIES • 47 G PROTEIN • 9 G CARBOHYDRATES • 12 G FAT

Scallops in Orange Sauce

RECOVERY

Scallops provide high-quality protein as well as omega-3 fatty acids and vitamin B$_{12}$, both of which boost cardiovascular health. For more recipes from Vincent Francoual, see pages 62, 90, and 188.

Makes 4 appetizer servings

PREP TIME: 15 MINUTES / COOK TIME: 40 MINUTES

2 leeks, tops and greens

10 fingerlings or small new potatoes (about 12 ounces)

1½ cups freshly squeezed orange juice

2 tablespoons chilled butter, diced into small pieces

2 teaspoons sherry vinegar or aged red wine vinegar

Salt and pepper

8 large sea scallops

1 cup all-purpose flour

2 tablespoons extra virgin olive oil

1 large orange, peeled and segmented

Preheat the oven to 400°F. Wash the leeks and potatoes. Cut the leeks into 2″ sticks, and slice the potatoes. Bring water to a boil in a medium pot. Season with salt and add the leeks to the pot. Cook the leeks until tender, about 10 to 12 minutes. Use the same technique in another pot for the potatoes, cooking for about 10 minutes or until tender. Add the orange juice to a medium saucepan and bring to a boil, reducing the juice until it's the texture of syrup, about 15 to 20 minutes. Whisk in the diced butter until it's well incorporated, then add the vinegar.

To sear the scallops, season them with salt and pepper and coat both sides in the flour. Heat a sauté pan with the olive oil on medium-high heat. When the oil is hot, add the scallops to the pan (do not overcrowd the pan) and place the pan in the oven. Cook for about 4 minutes, remove the pan from the oven, and immediately place it on a medium-heat burner. Flip the scallops and sear for another minute.

To serve, warm the vegetable garnish and place it in the center of a plate. Top with the scallops and add the orange segments. Drizzle the sauce around the garnish.

PER SERVING: 234 CALORIES • 9 G PROTEIN • 37 G CARBOHYDRATES • 6 G FAT

Shrimp Scampi

"Quick and easy to make, these sautéed jumbo shrimp are a real crowd-pleaser," Paul Raftis says. Shrimp are a good low-calorie, low-fat source of protein. They also provide cancer-fighting selenium, bone-building vitamin D, heart-healthy vitamin B$_{12}$, and omega-3 fatty acids, which benefit cardiovascular health. For more from Paul Raftis, see page 84.

Makes 4 servings

PREP TIME: 15 MINUTES / COOK TIME: 10–15 MINUTES

- 1½ pounds shrimp (about 20–24 shrimp), peeled and deveined
- 1 teaspoon kosher salt
- 1 teaspoon ground black pepper
- 4 teaspoons extra-virgin olive oil
- 4 teaspoons unsalted butter
- 2 teaspoons chopped garlic
- 1⅓ cups white wine
- 4 teaspoons freshly squeezed lemon juice
- 4 teaspoons Dijon mustard

Season the shrimp with the salt and pepper. Heat the olive oil in a large, nonstick sauté pan over medium-high heat. Add the shrimp and cook, stirring frequently, for 3 to 4 minutes per side. Remove the shrimp from the pan.

To make the sauce, reduce the heat to medium and add the butter and garlic. Cook, stirring frequently, for 30 seconds. Add the white wine, lemon juice, and Dijon mustard. Reduce until thickened. Season to taste with salt and pepper. Add the shrimp to the sauce and keep warm.

To serve, put the shrimp on a warm dinner plate, pour the sauce over shrimp, and garnish with chopped parsley.

PER SERVING: 190 CALORIES • 7 G PROTEIN • 4 G CARBOHYDRATES • 9 G FAT

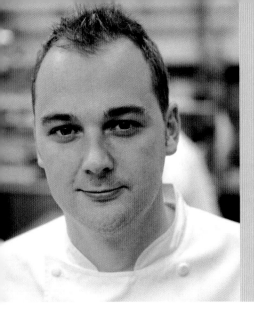

DANIEL HUMM

Daniel Humm was a competitive cyclist in Switzerland, where he grew up, but gave it up to pursue a career in the kitchen. "There were two or three other cyclists who always beat me," he says. "So I decided to cook, which I'd been doing since I was 14." Now he is the executive chef of New York City's Eleven Madison Park—and a runner. Humm trained for the ING New York City Marathon in 2008, adding as much as 30 miles a week to his usual weekly 45 miles. It paid off: The chef finished in 2:51, or 450th place, and rewarded himself with white truffles and a bottle of vintage Barolo. For more, go to elevenmadisonpark.com.

Shrimp with Israeli Couscous, Spring Peas, Mint, and Lemon

`TRAINING`

Israeli couscous, which is sometimes called pearl couscous because of its smooth, round shape, is a good source of carbohydrates. For more from Daniel Humm, see page 83.

Makes 6 servings

PREP TIME: 15 MINUTES / COOK TIME: 10 MINUTES

2 lemons

1 cup grated Parmesan cheese

2 cups almonds, blanched

3/4 cup + 2 teaspoons extra virgin olive oil

1 bunch mint leaves (about 1 cup)

1 pound Israeli couscous

1 pound large shrimp or prawns, cleaned, peeled, and deveined

2 cups fresh or frozen spring peas

2 tablespoons lemon juice, or to taste

Salt and ground red pepper, to taste

1 bunch mint leaves (for garnish)

1/2 cup toasted almonds (for garnish)

Zest and juice 1 lemon; reserve the zest. Make a pesto by combining the lemon juice, Parmesan cheese, almonds, 3/4 cup of the olive oil, and the mint. Boil liberally salted water in a large pot. Add the couscous and cook for 6 to 7 minutes. Drain and set aside. Heat a large skillet with the 2 teaspoons of olive oil. Add the shrimp and sauté quickly, about 3 to 4 minutes per side; add the peas and continue cooking. Add 1 cup of the pesto, followed by the couscous. Juice the second lemon and season the couscous with the lemon juice, salt, and ground red pepper. Finish with the mint leaves, reserved lemon zest, and almonds.

PER SERVING: 650 CALORIES • 32 G PROTEIN • 77 G CARBOHYDRATES • 24 G FAT

Spicy Salmon Lettuce "Gyros"

"This lower-carb version of a classic Greek gyro, where I substitute lettuce for a pita, is one of my favorite postrun meals because it's satisfying but still light and fresh," says Cat Cora, whose family is from Greece. Oily cold-water fish such as salmon contains omega-3 fatty acids, which benefit cardiovascular health. Look for wild-caught salmon for the biggest nutritional boost. For more from Cat Cora, see pages 20, 120, 155, 157, and 174.

Makes 4 servings

PREP TIME: 10 MINUTES / COOK TIME: 10 MINUTES

2 tablespoons olive oil+ additional for
 brushing

Juice of 2 limes

1 tablespoon chili powder

1 tablespoon ground cumin

1 teaspoon ground red pepper

1½ teaspoons sea salt

¼ teaspoon freshly ground black pepper

5 (4 ounce) salmon fillets (can also use
 halibut, snapper, or branzino)

1 head butter lettuce

1 head radicchio

1 tomato, diced

1 onion, diced

½ cup prepared tzatziki (in the yogurt
 section of the supermarket)

¼ cup chopped scallions

Preheat the grill to 400°F. In a 13" × 9" baking dish, combine the olive oil, lime juice, chili powder, cumin, red pepper, sea salt, and black pepper. Add the fish fillets and turn them so every side is coated with marinade. Marinate for 10 minutes.

Form lettuce cups by gently separating the heads of the butter lettuce and radicchio. Line a whole leaf of butter lettuce with radicchio.

Brush the fillets with olive oil before placing them on the grill. Cook on each side until the fish is opaque (cooking time will vary, depending on the thickness of the fillets, about 3 to 10 minutes). The fish should be firm to the touch, flaking easily.

Flake a generous amount of fish into each lettuce cup, or cut the fish into small chunks and place them in each cup. Top each cup with tomato and onion. Drizzle with the tzatziki, then garnish with the scallions. To eat, use a knife and fork, or eat it like a taco (a bit messier).

PER SERVING: 350 CALORIES • 31 G PROTEIN • 9 G CARBOHYDRATES • 22 G FAT

Tilapia with Papaya Ginger Relish and Summer Squash

Because of its high fat content, tilapia, even though it is a freshwater fish, is a good source of omega-3 fatty acids, which raise levels of high-density lipoprotein (HDL or "good" cholesterol). A sustainably farmed fish with easily renewed stocks, tilapia also provides potassium, which is important for electrolyte balance and regulating blood pressure. An aid to digestion, papayas have more vitamin C and potassium than oranges—and fewer calories. Find fish sauce and Thai bird's eye chili (an especially spicy variety) at Asian groceries or gourmet markets. For more from Simpson Wong, see page 158.

Makes 4 servings

PREP TIME: 20 MINUTES / COOK TIME: 25 MINUTES

Relish

¼ cup finely diced green mango

¼ cup finely diced semiripe papaya

1 tablespoon minced ginger

1 tablespoon minced garlic

1 tablespoon minced shallots

3 tablespoons fish sauce (available at Asian groceries)

4 tablespoons freshly squeezed lime juice

2 tablespoons sugar

1 Thai bird's eye chili, thinly sliced, or 1 tablespoon chili paste (optional)

¼ cup loosely packed julienned mint

¼ cup extra virgin olive oil

Salt and pepper to taste

"Salad"

2 tablespoons extra virgin olive oil

1 teaspoon minced garlic

2 summer squash such as lita squash or yellow squash (about 1 pound)

2 radishes, thinly sliced

4 roasted golden beets, quartered

1 zucchini, thinly sliced

Salt and pepper to taste

Fish

4 tilapia fillets (6 ounces each)

Salt and pepper to taste

2 tablespoons extra virgin olive oil

Relish

Mix together the mango, papaya, ginger, garlic, shallots, fish sauce, lime juice, sugar, and chili. Set aside.

Drizzle with olive oil. Season with salt and pepper.

(continued on page 148)

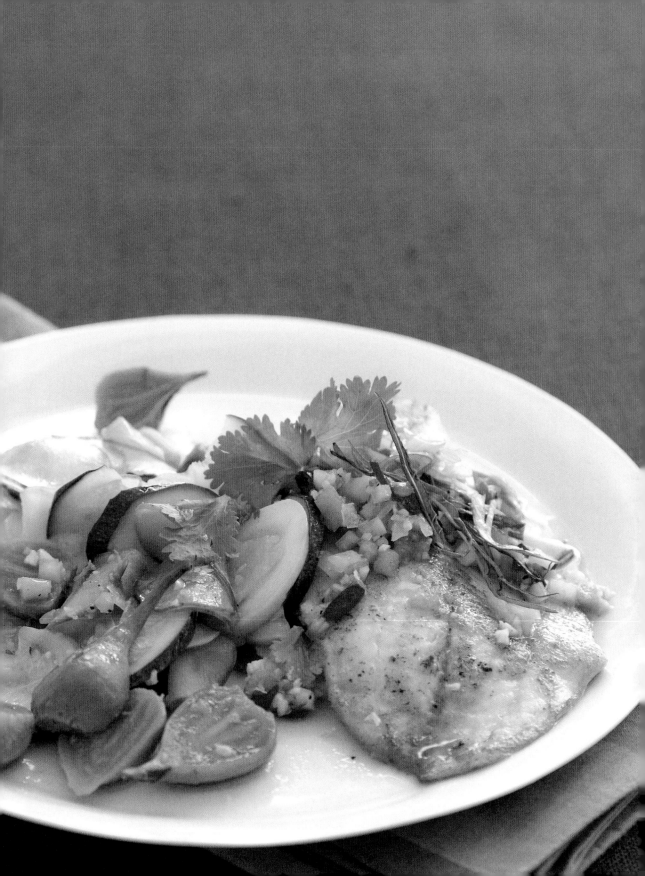

Squash

Heat the olive oil in a large saucepan over medium heat. Add the garlic and cook, stirring frequently, for about 2 minutes or until fragrant. Add the summer squash, radishes, golden beets, and zucchini, and cook until golden-brown, about 5 minutes. Season with salt and pepper.

Fish

Season the tilapia with the salt and pepper. While sautéing the "salad," heat the olive oil in a large size skillet over medium heat. Add the fish skin-side down and cook until the skin turns crispy, about 3 minutes. Then flip the fish and continue cooking for about 2 minutes, or until the fish flakes easily.

Divide the "salad" among 4 plates, top each with a fish fillet and relish.

PER SERVING: 390 CALORIES • 38 G PROTEIN • 20 G CARBOHYDRATES • 18 G FAT

BOBBY FLAY

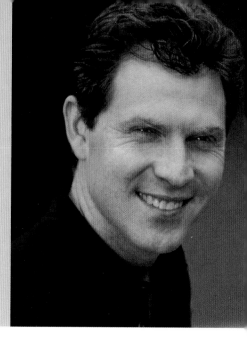

Even though he stars in the Food Network show *Boy Meets Grill* and pens cookbooks about grilling, don't expect Bobby Flay to celebrate the completion of a long race with a big barbecue meal. "That was a gigantic mistake," says Flay, referring to his postrace fuel after finishing the 2002 New York City Marathon. "It made me nauseated." A distance runner in high school, the native New Yorker reached for an apple when he ran New York in 2006, but admits he craves a classic banana split as an after-race indulgence. "My diet is simple. I just eat whatever I feel like eating," Flay says. "As long as it tastes good, it doesn't matter what's in a dish." For more, go to bobbyflay.com.

Beef and Sun-Dried Tomato Flatbread Pizza

TRAINING

Bobby Flay makes his own flatbread dough but says it's fine to buy premade pizza dough to use on the grill or whole wheat pitas. Beef packs in protein, which is necessary to jump-start muscle repair after a race, while the bread, beans, and vegetables provide carbs and fiber. For more from Bobby Flay, see page 87.

Makes 8 servings

PREP TIME: 20 MINUTES + 4 HOURS MARINATING TIME / COOK TIME: 15 MINUTES

8 whole wheat pitas (6" in diameter) or
    16–20 ounces of fresh or refrigerated
    pizza dough
1 beef tenderloin (8 ounces)
1 head garlic + 2 cloves garlic, smashed
½ cup + 4 tablespoons olive oil
1 cup cooked white beans
1 tablespoon freshly squeezed lemon juice

1 tablespoon fresh thyme
Salt and freshly ground pepper to taste
6 sun-dried tomatoes in oil, drained and
    julienned
4 roasted shallots, thinly sliced
1 tablespoon balsamic vinegar
1 teaspoon honey

(continued on page 151)

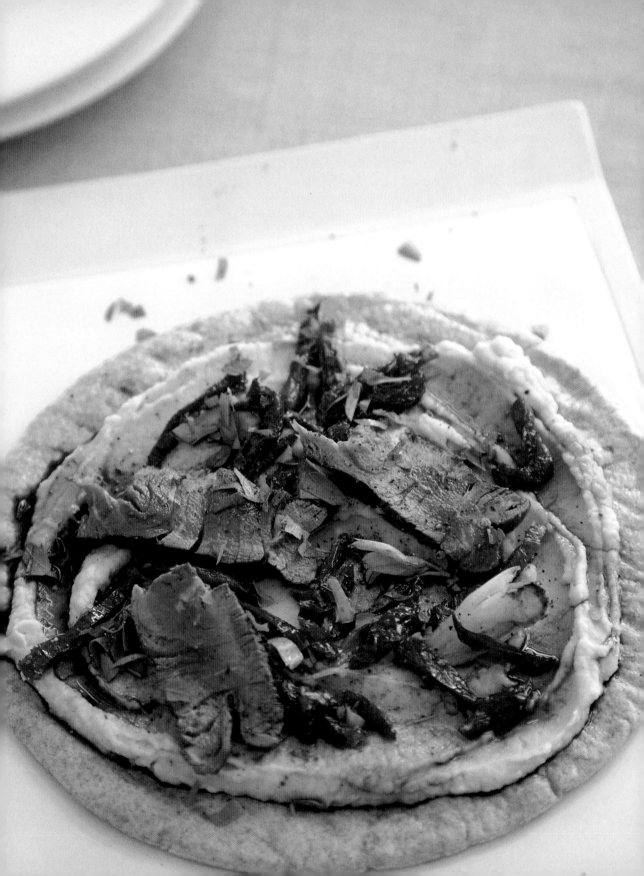

Marinate the beef with the head of garlic in $\frac{1}{2}$ cup of the olive oil for 4 hours or overnight. Coat the grill rack with cooking spray and preheat the grill. Cook the tenderloin on high heat on both sides for about 4 minutes on each side, or until a thermometer inserted in the center registers 145°F for medium rare. Let the tenderloin rest for 10 minutes, then thinly slice.

Puree the beans, 2 tablespoons of the olive oil, 2 remaining garlic cloves, lemon juice, and thyme in a food processor until smooth. Season with salt and pepper to taste. Mix together the tomatoes, shallots, remaining 2 tablespoons of olive oil, vinegar, and honey.

Divide the pizza dough into quarters and roll out on a lightly floured surface until thin but still stretchy. Roll into 6″ rounds or squares.

Brush the dough (or pitas if using) with olive oil, season with salt and pepper, and grill each side until golden (about 1 minute) over medium-high heat.

Spread each flatbread or pita with a thin layer of white bean puree, sliced beef, and tomato chutney. Serve immediately.

USING WHOLE-WHEAT PITA:
PER SERVING: 460 CALORIES • 16 G PROTEIN • 48 G CARBOHYDRATES • 24 G FAT

Naan Pizza with Canadian Bacon, Asparagus, and Fontina Cheese

Pam Anderson uses naan, an Indian flatbread, as the base for this pizza topped with pesto and Canadian bacon. One cup of asparagus contains about a third of the Daily Value for vitamin C. It is also a good source of vitamin K, which is important for bone health and blood clotting. The cheeses contain calcium; 1 serving of the pizza provides 30 percent of the Daily Value for calcium, which you can boost by sprinkling Parmesan cheese over the hot pizza. For more from Pam Anderson, see pages 30 and 98.

Makes 4 servings

PREP TIME: 10 MINUTES / COOK TIME: 15 MINUTES

2 (9") naan (8-ounce package)

$\frac{1}{3}$ cup part-skim ricotta cheese

$\frac{1}{4}$ cup prepared pesto

8 asparagus spears, tough ends snapped off, cut into $1\frac{1}{2}$" lengths

1 teaspoon extra-virgin olive oil

Salt and ground black pepper to taste

3 slices Canadian bacon, cut into thin strips

$\frac{2}{3}$ cup (2 ounces) grated fontina cheese

Adjust an oven rack to the lower-middle position and heat the oven to 425°F. Place the flatbreads on a baking sheet. Mix the ricotta and pesto and dollop onto the breads. Toss the asparagus with the oil and a light sprinkling of salt and pepper. Evenly distribute the spears, along with the Canadian bacon, over the naan. Bake until the breads are warm throughout and the asparagus is bright green, about 10 minutes. Remove them from the oven. Divide the fontina equally and top each naan with a portion of cheese. Return them to the oven and continue to bake until the breads are crisp and the cheese has melted, about 5 minutes longer. Cut each naan into quarters, serving each person 2 slices, or half a naan.

PER SERVING: 360 CALORIES • 18 G PROTEIN • 32 G CARBOHYDRATES • 18 G FAT

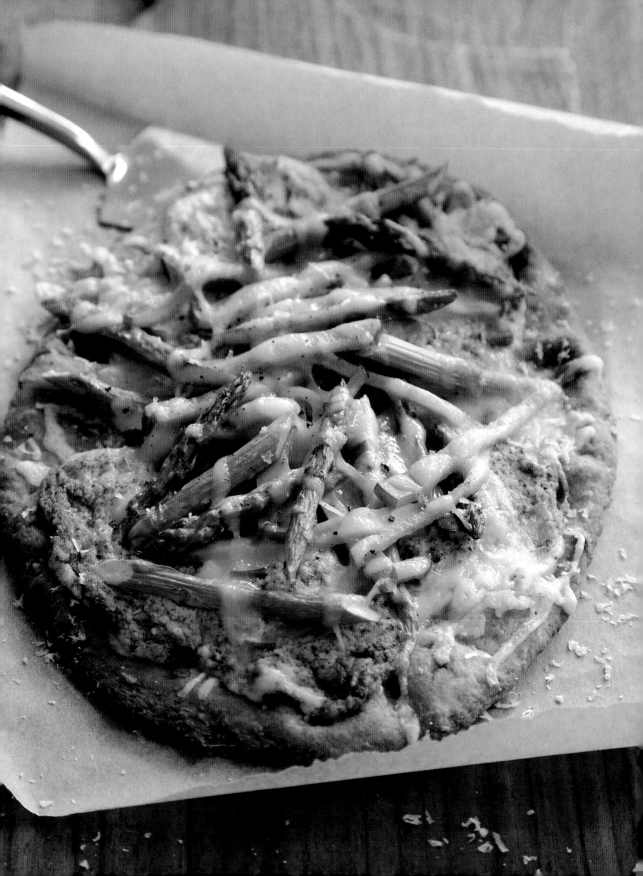

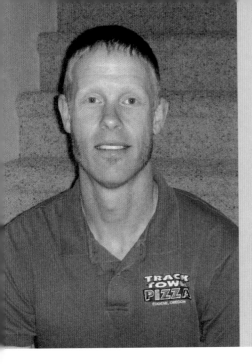

MIKE RIPLEY

Mike Ripley's Track Town Pizza has been the runners' hangout in Eugene, Oregon, for 30 years. The restaurant walls display photos of local track legends, such as Steve Prefontaine, Alberto Salazar, and Mary Decker Slaney, while more recent regulars include Olympians Dathan Ritzenhein and Marla Runyan. Menu item names reflect Ripley's own background as a longtime runner and track-and-field fan. Besides the Triple Jump Pizza, there's the all-meat Heptathlon and the vegetarian Pole Vault. When the 2008 U.S. Olympic Track and Field Trials were held over 10 days at the University of Oregon's Hayward Field, less than a mile away, the pizzeria sold 3,000 pies. "The orders were manageable," Ripley says, "like a nice tempo run." For more, go to tracktownpizza.com.

Triple Jump Pizza   `TRAINING`

"The blend of cheeses and spices in this pizza takes a detour from the traditional red-sauce pizza," Ripley says. *The cheeses provide calcium, while the vitamins, antioxidants, and other nutrients in spinach have been shown to protect against heart disease, osteoporosis, arthritis, and some cancers.*

Makes 6 slices

PREP TIME: 10 MINUTES / COOK TIME: 10 MINUTES

10 ounces prepared pizza dough

1 tablespoon extra virgin olive oil

1 teaspoon minced fresh garlic

1 cup (4 ounces) fresh spinach

2 cups (5 ounces) grated mozzarella cheese

¼ cup (1 ounce) grated provolone cheese

2 ounces feta cheese

1 small red onion, thinly sliced

3 ounces fresh, spicy sausage, browned and sliced into nickel-size pieces

Preheat oven to 425°F. Stretch the dough to a 12"-diameter round and use a fork to perforate the dough over the entire surface to prevent bubbles while cooking. Spread the olive oil over the entire dough round with a pastry brush. Spread the garlic over the dough. Place the spinach on top of the crust. Mix together the mozzarella and provolone cheeses, then sprinkle over the spinach. Crumble the feta onto the pizza, then sprinkle the onions onto the pizza. Place the spicy sausage on top. Bake in the oven for 10 minutes, or until the cheese is melted and the sausage is heated through.

PER SERVING: 250 CALORIES • 14 G PROTEIN • 23 G CARBOHYDRATES • 13 G FAT

Basque Grilled Vegetable Kebabs with Key Lime Chimichurri

One of Cat Cora's simple tricks to add taste without calories is to use vinegars and citrus juices, as in these vegetable kebabs flavored with a Basque-style green sauce. "When you put a squeeze of citrus—lemon or lime—on anything, it just makes it pop," she says. For more from Cat Cora, see pages 20, 120, 155, 157, and 174.

Makes 4 servings

PREP TIME: 15 MINUTES / COOK TIME: 10 MINUTES

Kebabs

3 bell peppers, all colors, cut into 2" pieces

2 portobello mushrooms, quartered

2 zucchini, cut into 2" rounds

1 red onion, cut in 2" pieces

Vegetable Rub

Salt and freshly ground black pepper

½ tablespoon chili powder

1 teaspoon sea salt

1 tablespoon dried orange rind

Basque-Style Green Sauce

6 garlic cloves, chopped

3 dried bay leaves

1 fresh poblano pepper, coarsely chopped with the seeds left in (optional)

1 fresh serrano chile, coarsely chopped with the seeds left in (optional)

½ tablespoon sea salt

⅓ cup finely chopped, fresh Italian flat-leaf parsley

¼ cup finely chopped, fresh oregano

½ cup finely chopped, fresh basil

3 Key limes (or 6 teaspoons bottled Key lime juice)

⅓ cup olive oil

(continued)

Rub

Combine the table salt, pepper, chili powder, sea salt, and orange rind. Cover the bell peppers, mushrooms, zucchini, and onion with the rub and let them rest in a baking dish or large bowl.

Green Sauce

Combine the garlic, bay leaves, peppers, and sea salt in a mortar and mash with a pestle until a smooth paste is formed. (If you don't have a mortar and pestle, put all the ingredients in a blender along with just a teaspoon or so of vinegar.) Transfer to a mixing bowl and add the parsley, oregano, and basil. Juice the key limes into the bowl. Whisk in the olive oil until well combined. Set aside.

Grilled Vegetables

Coat the grill rack with cooking spray, and preheat the grill. Skewer the veggies and grill on all sides for about 8 minutes. Serve over a bed of steamed brown rice and drizzle the sauce over the skewered vegetables.

PER SERVING: 220 CALORIES • 7 G PROTEIN • 29 G CARBOHYDRATES • 11 G FAT

Curried Lentils with Butternut Squash

"For such a homey, healthy dish, this dinner has a lot of pizzazz, thanks to the fresh ginger, curry, and chili powder," says Cat Cora. In her cookbook Cooking from the Hip, *she focuses on fast, healthy recipes that are easy to prepare. Since you can cook the lentils and chunks of squash beforehand and keep them in the fridge overnight, the final prep time for this recipe is minimal. Plus, you can peel the fresh gingerroot quickly by scraping it with a spoon.*

Cora likes to serve this dinner with fresh mango chutney and a big bowl of brown rice. Lentils are a low-calorie, low-fat source of cholesterol-reducing fiber, as well as protein, B vitamins, iron, and other minerals. They also cook more quickly than other legumes. Butternut squash contains potassium, fiber, and the antioxidant beta carotene. For more from Cat Cora, see pages 20, 120, 155, and 174.

Makes 2 servings as a hearty main dish or 4 as a side dish

PREP TIME: 15 MINUTES / COOK TIME: 20–30 MINUTES

- 1 cup dry lentils
- 1 small butternut squash, cut into 2" × 2" pieces with skin on
- 1 tablespoon extra virgin olive oil
- 1 tablespoon curry powder
- 1 teaspoon grated fresh gingerroot
- 1 teaspoon chili powder
- Salt and pepper to taste
- ¼ cup shredded coconut (optional)

Spray a 2-quart baking dish with cooking spray and set aside. Pour the lentils into a deep pot and cover with cold water. Bring the water to a boil, reduce the heat, and add squash pieces (leave the skin on to add nutrients and texture to the dish). Simmer until the squash is soft (about 1 hour). Remove the pot from the heat, drain, and set aside. With tongs, pull out the chunks of squash and mash them roughly, skins and all, with a fork, ricer, or potato masher.

Preheat the oven to 400°F. Mix the drained, cooked lentils and mashed squash with the olive oil, curry powder, gingerroot, chili powder, salt, and pepper in a large bowl. Spoon the mixture into the baking dish. At this point, you can cover the dish and refrigerate it for a few hours or even overnight. Bake 20 minutes or 25 to 30 minutes if it's been refrigerated. Serve warm, garnished with shredded coconut.

PER SERVING: 530 CALORIES • 32 G PROTEIN • 94 G CARBOHYDRATES • 8 G FAT

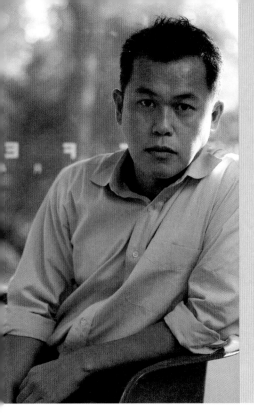

SIMPSON WONG

The date was Friday the 13th when Simpson Wong felt a tightness in his chest and left arm while lifting weights at the gym. The Malaysian-born chef thought he had heartburn but hours later discovered he'd had a heart attack. It was a wake-up call. "I looked young, I ran, I wasn't fat," Wong says. "But I smoked, and my family has a history of heart problems." He also realized that his role as chef-owner of a New York City restaurant meant he consumed nearly 2 cups of butter a night, while tasting dishes during dinner service. He quit smoking, overhauled the menu to reduce butter and cream, and continued running five times a week, 40 to 50 minutes at a time, sometimes twice a day. The regimen so far is working. "My cardiologist thinks I'm such a model patient that she wants me to talk to her other patients," Wong says. "Besides eliminating most fat, I eat normally—and a lot." For more, go to cafesean.com.

Eggplant Sandwich

`RECOVERY`

This eggplant dish is dressed with a vinaigrette flavored with fresh sawtooth, an herb that tastes like cilantro crossed with basil. You can find it at specialty Asian markets, or use fresh basil as a substitute. The roasted red bell peppers provide plenty of vitamin C, and the eggplant has fiber. Best of all, most of the fat in the dish comes from grapeseed oil, which contains the antioxidant vitamin E and polyunsaturated fats that reduce blood cholesterol levels. For more recipes from Simpson Wong, see page 146.

Makes 4 servings

PREP TIME: 20 MINUTES / COOK TIME: 25 MINUTES

Vinaigrette

½ cup fresh sawtooth

1½ teaspoons freshly squeezed lemon juice

½ teaspoon salt

Ground red pepper to taste

½ teaspoon sugar

4 tablespoons grapeseed or canola oil

Salt and pepper to taste

Eggplant

  2 Japanese or baby eggplants, halved

  3 tablespoons extra virgin olive oil

  Salt and pepper

  4 tablespoons soft feta cheese

  2 medium red bell peppers, roasted, peeled, and seeded

  1 cup arugula

Preheat the overn to 375°F. Puree the sawtooth, lemon juice, salt, red pepper, sugar, and grapeseed oil in a blender until smooth. Season with salt and pepper to taste and set aside.

Lightly score the inside of the halved eggplants, drizzle them with the olive oil, and lay them skin-side down on a baking sheet. Sprinkle with more olive oil and roast for 20 to 25 minutes.

Place the eggplant halves face-up on 4 serving plates, season them with salt and pepper, and divide the feta cheese, roasted pepper, and arugula among the 4 halves. Drizzle with vinaigrette (you may have some left over).

Serve and eat open-faced.

PER SERVING: 548 CALORIES • 6 G PROTEIN • 16 G CARBOHYDRATES • 52 G FAT

Panini with Brie, Chocolate, and Olives

Tuesday Evans says this unusual combination came about one night when she and her husband were snacking on cheese along with leftover torte. "The combination of the sweet, salt, tangy, earthy flavors mixed with the smooth texture of the torte and brie is just amazing," she says. For more from Tuesday Evans, see pages 168 and 185.

Makes 2 servings

PREP TIME: 10 MINUTES / COOK TIME: 4 MINUTES

4 slices ciabatta or sourdough bread

1 teaspoon olive oil

2–4 slices of Brie (about 3 ounces or more, to taste)

2 tablespoons semisweet chocolate chips

1–2 tablespoons mixed, pitted olives

Brush both sides of the bread with olive oil and grill in a panini maker until they start to turn golden-brown, about 2 minutes. Place the cheese on 1 slice of the bread and sprinkle sparingly with some diced olives, then top with some chocolate chips (to taste). Top with the other slice of the bread and then grill more on each side until the cheese and chocolate are melted, another minute or 2.

Alternatively, simply assemble sandwich and toast in a skillet as you would a basic grilled cheese sandwich, flipping halfway through.

PER SERVING: 590 CALORIES • 24 G PROTEIN • 79 G CARBOHYDRATES • 20 G FAT

ROLF RUNKEL

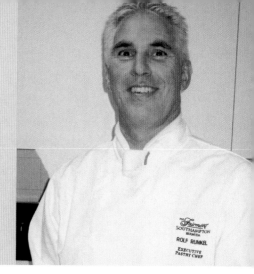

As the executive pastry chef at the Ritz-Carlton in Grand Cayman, Rolf Runkel spends his days making such calorie-laden indulgences as white chocolate and passion fruit cake and apple tarte tatin. But after a day surrounded by sweets, he takes in the ocean sunsets on runs of 8 to 12 miles, 5 days a week. He is a regular at local half and full marathons and finished ninth in a local triathlon. For more, go to ritzcarlton.com.

Tortilla Pie

`TRAINING`

This spicy, multilayered tortilla-and-bean pie is one of Runkel's favorite postrun meals. "The pie is high in carbs, includes protein, and is great hot or cold," he says. It contains plenty of fiber, which benefits the heart and helps fill you up. For more from Rolf Runkel, see page 22.

Makes 6 servings

PREP TIME: 10 MINUTES / COOK TIME: 45 MINUTES

1 tablespoon olive oil

1 medium onion, chopped

½ cup chopped celery

1 clove garlic, minced

1 can (15 ounces) yellow corn, drained

1 can (15 ounces) kidney beans, drained

1 can (15 ounces) black beans, drained

1 can (15 ounces) white beans, drained

1 can (6 ounces) tomato paste

1 tablespoon taco seasoning

5 soft tortillas (10"–12" each)

1 cup shredded Cheddar cheese

Preheat the oven to 350°F. Heat the oil in a large skillet over medium heat and add the onions, celery, and garlic. Cook, stirring frequently, for 5 minutes until the onions are golden. Add the corn, kidney beans, black beans, white beans, tomato paste, and seasoning, and heat thoroughly. Set 2 tablespoons of the bean mix aside. Place 1 tortilla on a baking sheet lightly coated with cooking spray, and spoon a few tablespoons of the bean mix onto it; spread evenly. Place a tortilla on top of beans, top with the mix again, and repeat until pie is 5 layers high. Add 2 tablespoons of water to the remaining mix and spread it over the top of the tortilla (this will prevent it from drying out during baking). Bake for 35 minutes. Sprinkle with the Cheddar, and bake until the cheese is melted. Let it sit for 15 minutes, then serve.

PER SERVING: 470 CALORIES • 22 G PROTEIN • 77 G CARBOHYDRATES • 12 G FAT

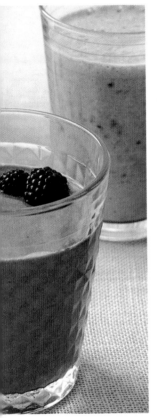

Beverages

Every athlete knows that water is the perfect beverage for staying hydrated. It's convenient, calorie free, and—when it comes from the tap—cheap. Still, it's worth noting that plain water won't do anything to replenish critical nutrients you need after a good workout. That's why sports drinks such as Gatorade are popular—because they replace spent carbohydrates, protein, and electrolytes.

Still, sometimes you want a bit more bang from your beverage, and even athletes can't stomach sports drinks all the time. Our running chefs have devised creative ways to feed your thirst while bolstering supplies of the nutrients your body needs. Plus, they taste great.

After a workout, "Iron Chef" Cat Cora likes to make a Seasonal Fruit Smoothie using whatever seasonal fruit she's got on hand. The smoothie replenishes energy with carbs in the form of quickly absorbed fruit sugars, plus protein from yogurt, soy milk, and almonds. The go-to beverage for chef Richard Sandoval, who is based in L.A., is a simple, refreshing agua fresca. It is literally "fresh water"—no more than water blended with vegetables or fruit with a little sugar.

In addition to the quick energy lift of sugar, caffeine is also a favorite energizer, either before or after a workout. Research has consistently shown that caffeine boosts endurance and speed. Artisanal coffee-shop owner Gabrielle Rubinstein cools down after warm-weather runs with her shop's signature iced coffee. And at mile 20 of the New York City Marathon, which is held each November, chocolatier Jacques Torres refueled with a nontraditional race refresher: his famous hot chocolate.

All-Natural Protein Shake

Chocolate-Espresso Smoothie

Coffee Granita

Chocorange Creamsicle

Dos Aguas Frescas

Jacques Torres's Hot Chocolate

Joe's Iced Coffee

Paley's Energy Drink

Seasonal Fruit Smoothie

All-Natural Protein Shake

Instead of protein powder, the protein in this shake comes from pasteurized egg whites, which are available in cartons in the dairy case. Cliff Pleau suggests making this shake before your morning run, and then drinking it within 20 minutes after your workout to speed muscle recovery. "You can use most any kind of fruit you have on hand," he says. "I use whatever is left over from my children's breakfasts." You can adjust the liquid measurements to desired taste and consistency. For more from Cliff Pleau, see page 59.

Makes 1 serving

PREP TIME: 10 MINUTES

1 very ripe banana, fresh or frozen, peeled and cut in chunks

½ cup fresh or frozen fruit (berries, melon, mango, pineapple, etc.)

⅓ cup light vanilla soy milk

⅓ cup egg whites, pasteurized

⅓ cup plain low-fat yogurt

Orange juice, pure vanilla extract, flax seed, wheat germ (optional)

Add the banana, fruits, soy milk, egg whites, yogurt, and any of the optional ingredients to a blender cup. Puree until the mixture is smooth and serve.

PER SERVING: 256 CALORIES • 15 G PROTEIN • 46 G CARBOHYDRATES • 3 G FAT

DAVID CHESAREK

Pastry chef David Chesarek is a chocoholic so dedicated that he eats the sweet stuff even after a run—although he learned the hard way not to reach for something too rich. "Pounding brownies after a run isn't smart, trust me," says Chesarek, who earned his baking stripes at restaurants in New York City and San Francisco, where he also ran his own bakery. A former hurdler who qualified for the 1988 Olympic Trials, the California native now coaches track part-time at Los Gatos High School, near where he lives in San Jose. He still enjoys post-workout smoothies, a habit he developed while a student at UC Berkeley. "It became my way to reward myself after a run," Chesarek says. "Great smoothies, like great cakes, are all about quality ingredients." For more, go to SacherDad.com.

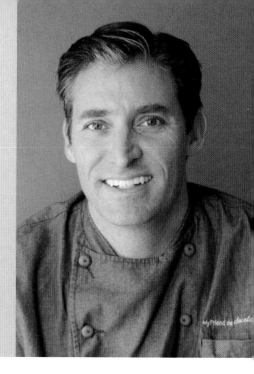

Chocolate-Espresso Smoothie

QUICK AND EASY   RECOVERY

David Chesarek gets his postworkout chocolate fix from this chocolate and banana smoothie spiked with espresso. "It gets your blood sugar up and rehydrates," he says. Chocolate milk has an optimum carbs-to-protein ratio that helps speed muscle recovery. The probiotics in yogurt give this drink an extra immunity boost, while the banana replenishes potassium, necessary for electrolyte and fluid balance in the body. Caffeine has been shown to boost athletic performance and endurance. For more from David Chesarek, see page 13.

Makes 2 servings

PREP TIME: 10 MINUTES

8 ounces (1 cup) chocolate yogurt, such as Brown Cow Cream Top

1 large banana, browned and frozen

2 shots espresso, chilled

2 cups ice (about 24 ice cubes)

12 chocolate-covered espresso beans

Place half of the yogurt, the banana, espresso, ice, and espresso beans in a blender and puree until smooth. Add the remaining yogurt and pulse until smooth. (If you add the full container of yogurt at the beginning, the mixture is too thick to blend easily.) For a thicker smoothie, blend in up to 1 cup more ice.

PER SERVING: 230 CALORIES • 7 G PROTEIN • 39 G CARBOHYDRATES • 7 G FAT

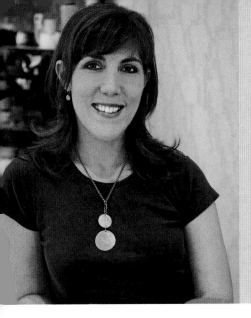

GABRIELLE RUBINSTEIN

Like many runners, Gabrielle Rubinstein relies on coffee to get going. So when she and her brother, Jonathan, opened a coffee spot called Joe in New York City, a ready group of caffeinated striders formed a running club. Team Joe meets at one of the café's five locations and its members run as little or as much as they want. "Afterward, I treat everyone to free coffee," says Rubinstein. Many of the runners have grown so addicted to the ritual that they've trained for and run the New York City Marathon together. For more, go to joetheartofcoffee.com.

Coffee Granita

QUICK AND EASY | TRAINING

Gabrielle Rubinstein and her brother and business partner, Jonathan, went to Rome on a coffee fact-finding mission a few years ago. They fell in love with granita, a crushed Italian ice drink that is cool and refreshing in warm weather but contains just a fraction of the calories of ice cream. "In Italy, the drink has bigger granules of ice, while the Joe version is smoother, closer to a Slushee," Rubinstein says. For more from Gabrielle Rubinstein, see page 172.

Makes 2 servings
PREP TIME: 10 MINUTES

2 ounces espresso or strong coffee

3 ounces 1% milk

1 ounce half-and-half

2 cups (about 2 dozen) ice cubes

1 ounce chocolate syrup or cocoa powder (optional)

Mix the espresso, milk, half-and-half, ice cubes, and chocolate syrup in a blender for 25 seconds, or until smooth. Serve immediately.

PER SERVING (WITH CHOCOLATE SYRUP): 90 CALORIES • 2 G PROTEIN • 15 G CARBOHYDRATES • 2 G FAT

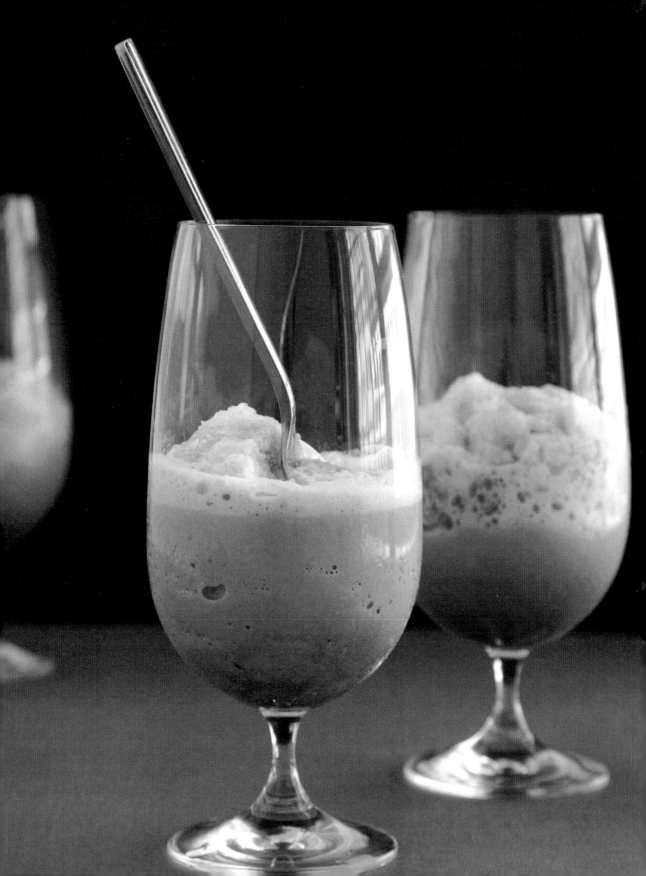

Chocorange Creamsicle

"This is a lightened, homemade version of an ice-cream truck Creamsicle but with chocolate in it," Tuesday Evans says. *Adjust the amount of ice cream depending on how thick you want the shake. One shake (half of this recipe) provides 110 percent of the Daily Value for vitamin C and 40 percent of the Daily Value for calcium. For more from Tuesday Evans, see pages 3, 160, and 185.*

Makes 2 servings

PREP TIME: 10 MINUTES

2 cups fat-free milk

2–4 scoops (1–2 cups) premium double-churned fat-free vanilla ice cream (such as Breyer's)

½ teaspoon pure vanilla extract

⅓ cup thawed pulp-free orange juice concentrate

2 tablespoons premium dark chocolate hot fudge sauce

Put milk, ice cream, vanilla extract, orange juice, and fudge sauce in a blender and mix until smooth.

PER SERVING (MADE WITH 2 SCOOPS ICE CREAM):
320 CALORIES • 13 G PROTEIN • 62 G CARBOHYDRATES • 3 G FAT

Dos Agua Frescas

Agua Fresca de Pepino (Cucumber Water)

These two nonalcoholic "fresh waters" are light and refreshing, blending fruit and vegetables with water. For more from Richard Sandoval, see pages 66 and 126.

Makes about 2 quarts

PREP TIME: 10 MINUTES

½ cup sugar, or to taste

1½ quarts water

3 large cucumbers, peeled and seeded

½ cup freshly squeezed lime juice

Dilute the sugar in 1 quart of the water.

Blend the cucumber, lime juice, and the rest of the water.

Mix both together and strain, if desired. Serve with a slice of cucumber on the rim.

PER SERVING: 60 CALORIES • 0 G PROTEIN • 15 G CARBOHYDRATES • 0 G FAT

Strawberry Pineapple Agua Fresca

Makes about 16 ounces

PREP TIME: 10 MINUTES

¼ cup chopped fresh pineapple

4 strawberries, hulled

1½ cups water

¼ cup sugar or to taste

Puree the pineapple and strawberries in a blender.

Strain the puree with a fine strainer to extract all of the juice. (You may need to add a little water.)

Combine the strained fruit puree and the water and add sugar to taste.

PER SERVING: 120 CALORIES • 0 G PROTEIN • 30 G CARBOHYDRATES • 0 G FAT

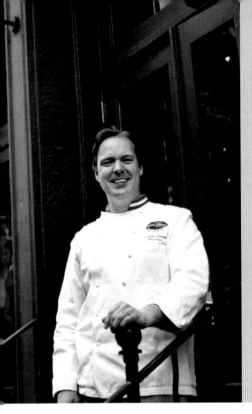

JACQUES TORRES

It is not surprising that a chocolatier who made his name from extravagant chocolate sculptures and handcrafted chocolate candies eschews water in favor of hot chocolate, even while running a race. At mile 20 of the New York City Marathon a few years ago, Jacques Torres enjoyed a mug of the sweet stuff, made from real chocolate, not cocoa powder, thanks to his girlfriend. "Once people could smell it, we shared everything we had," says Torres, who has run New York five times. The French-born chef often runs the 8 miles from his Manhattan home to his Brooklyn factory, a 7,500-square-foot space that churns out 60 to 70 tons of all-natural, preservative-free chocolate a year. At Torres's Manhattan shop, visitors can see how cocoa beans are processed into chocolate. While Torres doesn't snack on chocolate while running, it is part of his daily diet. "I taste a lot during recipe testing," he says. For more, go to jacquestorres.com.

Jacques Torres's Hot Chocolate

QUICK AND EASY   TRAINING

It's difficult to replicate Torres's famous hot chocolate without special kitchen equipment. This super-simple recipe is an adaptation. Dark chocolate contains antioxidant flavonoids, such as those found in red wine and green tea, which have been shown to decrease inflammation and high blood pressure.

Makes 1 serving

PREP TIME: 1 MINUTE / COOK TIME: 3–5 MINUTES

1 cup whole milk

2 ounces dark chocolate chips (cocoa content 60 percent or higher)

Heat the milk in a saucepan over medium heat. Add the chocolate chips. (You can use more than 2 ounces if you want a stronger flavor.) Stir until all of the chocolate melts and the mixture is blended. Pour into a mug and serve.

PER SERVING: 403 CALORIES • 10 G PROTEIN • 48 G CARBOHYDRATES • 22 G FAT

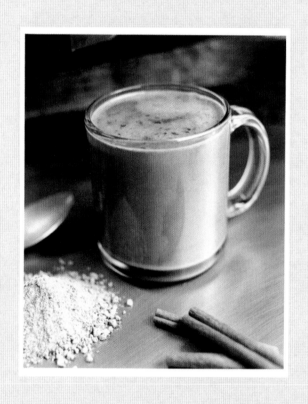

Joe's Iced Coffee

Simple syrup is a quick, easy way to sweeten drinks and eliminates the need to wait for sugar crystals to dissolve. For cold coffee drinks, use 1 part sugar to 1 part water. Bring the water and sugar to a boil, stir occasionally until the sugar is completely dissolved, then cool, bottle, and refrigerate. The syrup keeps for up to 3 months when stored in an airtight container and refrigerated. For more from Gabrielle Rubinstein, see page 166.

Makes 12 servings

PREP TIME: 10 MINUTES

½ pound very coarsely ground, medium-dark roast coffee

1 piece (1 foot square) cheesecloth

3 quarts cold water

Simple syrup, milk, chocolate syrup

Place the coffee in the piece of cheesecloth, tie it at the end, and submerge it in a container filled with the cold water. Let it stand overnight in the refrigerator. Remove the grind-filled cheesecloth and pour the coffee into 8-ounce glasses filled with ice.

PER SERVING (1 COFFEE WITH 3 TABLESPOONS SIMPLE SYRUP):
70 CALORIES • 0 G PROTEIN • 17 G CARBOHYDRATES • 0 G FAT

Paley's Energy Drink

The berries in this three-ingredient, all-natural drink provide carbohydrates and antioxidants. Vitaly Paley says this recipe fills one 16-ounce squeeze bottle to take along on a workout. Ginseng has been traditionally used as a stimulant and is said to improve energy, stamina, and alertness. For more from Vitaly Paley, see page 17.

Makes 1 serving

PREP TIME: 10 MINUTES

16 ounces purified water

2 teaspoons ginseng extract

1 handful seasonal berries (out of season, use $\frac{1}{2}$ cup frozen unsweetened berry puree)

Place the water, ginseng extract, and berries in a blender. Puree until smooth and strain if necessary. Will fill one 16-ounce squeeze bottle.

PER SERVING: 64 CALORIES • 1 G PROTEIN • 15 G CARBOHYDRATES • 1 G FAT

Seasonal Fruit Smoothie

You won't ever catch Cat Cora snacking on an energy bar. "Dried apricots and raisins mixed with almonds give me a lot of good energy," she says. The chef always includes protein in her snacks, like this seasonal fruit smoothie with its mix of low-fat yogurt, soy milk, and almonds, which satisfy hunger and promote muscle recovery. Almonds are an excellent source of the antioxidant vitamin E. Plus, the nut's monounsaturated fats benefit the heart. Soy is rich in heart-healthy omega-3 fatty acids, protein, vitamins, and minerals. For more from Cat Cora, see pages 20, 120, 145, 155, and 157.

Makes 2 servings

PREP TIME: 10 MINUTES

½ cup seasonal fruit (peaches, berries, and mango work well)

¾ cup plain low-fat yogurt

1 cup soy milk

6 almonds

1 tablespoon honey (optional)

Peel the fruit, if appropriate, and cut into small pieces. Put the fruit, yogurt, soy milk, almonds, and honey (if used) into a blender and puree until smooth. Pour the mixture into a chilled glass and serve with a straw. Add ice or use frozen fruit if you want to enjoy it really cold.

PER SERVING: 170 CALORIES • 12 G PROTEIN • 19 G CARBOHYDRATES • 6 G FAT

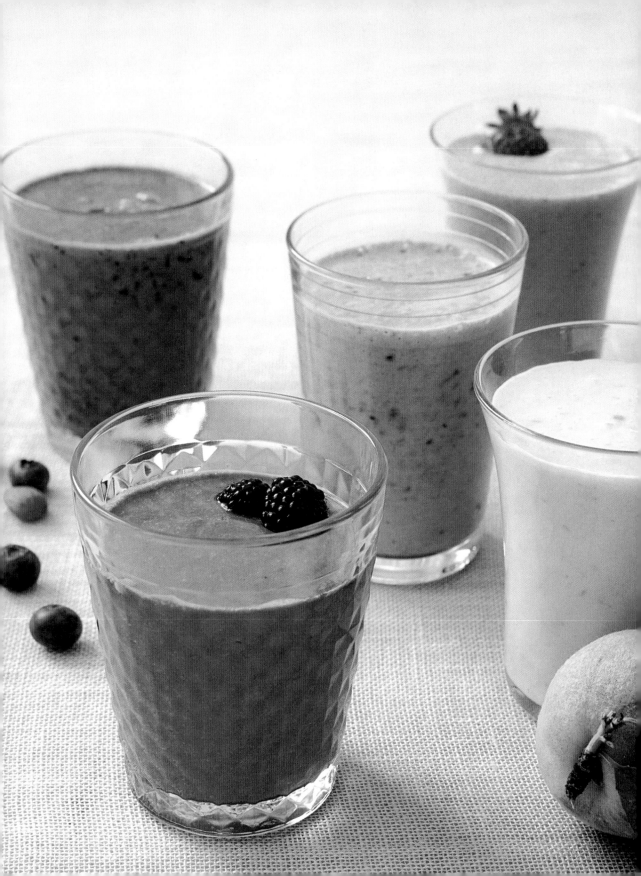

WINE

Studies have shown that a moderate drinking habit is better for your health than abstaining entirely from alcohol. Taken in moderation, alcohol benefits the heart and cardiovascular system and can help prevent type 2 diabetes and gallstones.

Researchers in Italy recently found that moderate drinking can actually help you live longer. Men who had up to four drinks a day (women up to two) cut their risk of death from any cause by 18 percent. The effect was pronounced no matter what kind of alcohol was consumed, be it beer, spirits, or wine. But keep in mind that to drink more than a moderate amount means the benefits are negated and alcohol becomes a toxin, not a tonic.

Red wine in particular has been shown to have additional healthful properties. The antioxidants and a substance called resveratrol in red wine have been linked to the prevention of blood vessel damage and blood clots. It also helps reduce inflammation (a common byproduct of exercise) and increases levels of high-density lipoprotein (HDL or "good") cholesterol.

Perhaps it's not surprising that studies also show that long-distance runners are more likely than couch potatoes to enjoy more than one glass of wine with dinner. The Marathon du Médoc in France's Bordeaux region fills its 8,500 spots well in advance of the September date of the race each year. The race's aid stations serve top wines from the famous wine-producing region (along with water), and winners take home their weight in grand crus.

Here in the United States, master sommeliers Andrea Immer Robinson, who lives in Napa Valley, and Bobby Stuckey, a Colorado resident, know the agonies of the finish line and an empty bottle of wine. Nearly 2 decades ago, when Robinson, then a financial analyst, decided to devote her career to understanding wine, she used running as a means to that end. Robinson spent 7 months exploring French and Italian wineries by Eurorail and hitchhiking. Every time she arrived somewhere new, she put on her sneakers and ran to various nearby vineyards. "I got to see what I couldn't by train," says Robinson, the author of an annual wine guide and other books about wine. "Then I'd meet winemakers who'd say, 'Didn't I see you running?' People thought I was nuts."

Winemakers in Friuli-Venezia Giulia, Italy, are no strangers to American runners. Each year Stuckey and his restaurant partner, Chef Lachlan Mackinnon-Patterson, take the staff from Frasca Food and Wine, their Boulder restaurant, to the northeastern region. Between trying new dishes and vintages for Frasca—which exclusively focuses on food and wine from Friuli—they do group runs among the grapes and in the foothills of the Alps.

Having worked with two staffers nationally ranked in trail running, Stuckey says, "It's easy to find people to run with, even if they're all better than me." The sommelier is no slouch himself. He finished the 2008 New York City Marathon in 2:45. He has also run Colorado's infamous Imogene Pass Run more than 10 times. Stuckey says completing the 17.1-mile slog across the San Juan Mountains and over the 13,120-foot summit "pulls me through the whole year."

When it comes to pairing wines with food, Robinson and Stuckey are not necessarily traditionalists.

"You don't need to drink white wine with fish or red wine with steak. An oak-aged Chardonnay can be eaten with steak if you want because it's heavier and richer than, say, a light Pinot Grigio," Robinson says. Lighter reds also work with red and white meats, she says, suggesting a Zinfandel with cured meats, baked ham, or pork loin. "As a rule of thumb, forget the color and pair a heavy dish with an intense wine and lighter fare with lighter wine," she says.

Stuckey agrees. He likes to drink such reds as Pinot Noir, grenache, or even a softer Barbaresco with seafood such as salmon and tuna. Reds are also a natural for pastas with red sauces.

"Sangiovese has a bright acidity that really works well with tomatoes," he says.

Light meats and whites are a good combination, he adds, such as Pinot Grigio with a turkey sandwich. "It's wonderful because of its melon and peach notes and aromas. It's not heavy with wood," Stuckey says. "One of my favorite pairings is dry Riesling with pork. It's a no-brainer." He also likes Riesling with a chicken stir-fry.

As for dessert? Robinson and Stuckey both like bubblies. Robinson says white sparkling wine has the right balance of acidity and sugar for fruit desserts such as pumpkin and apple pies. If chocolate is on the menu, Stuckey prefers red sparkling wines, which are typically lower in alcohol and have a soft sweetness.

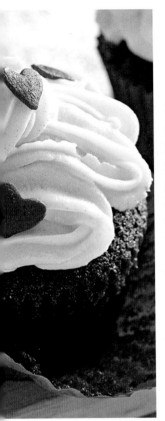

Desserts

Dessert is why we tack on another 5 miles to our long 10-miler, or bike a century instead of just a half. The good news is that a sweet such as dark chocolate has proven healthful properties, such as reducing inflammation from exercise and lowering high blood pressure. No wonder half the recipes feature it as an ingredient, as in Las Vegas pastry chef Megan Romano's Flourless Chocolate Cake or the chocolate sauce that Minneapolis chef Vincent Francoual, a native of France, likes with his Madeleines. The cocoa in New York City pastry chefs Beth Pilar and Ellen Sternau's recipe for Red Velvet Cupcakes provides not only color but also heart-healthy antioxidants.

Fresh fruit remains the simple, healthy way to end a meal, but that doesn't mean it has to be boring. Cookbook author Devin Alexander lightens the fat but not the flavor in her Roasted Pineapple à la Mode, and New York City restaurateur Joe Bastianich enjoys strawberries the classic Italian way: with balsamic vinegar and just a touch of sugar.

Chocolate-Dipped Strawberries

Chocolate, Fig, and Almond Bites

Chocolate-Hazelnut and Goat Cheese Melt

Finishing Kick Chocolate Sauce

Flourless Chocolate Cake

Madeleines

Red Velvet Cupcakes

Roasted Pineapple à la Mode

Strawberries with Balsamic Vinegar

Watermelon-Cantaloupe Salad

Chocolate-Dipped Strawberries

Unlike most chocolate, dark chocolate is rich in antioxidant polyphenols such as epicatechin, which is also found in green tea and red wine. Polyphenols help reduce high blood pressure and inflammation.

Research has shown that a mere 30 calories a day of dark chocolate results in a small but significant reduction in blood pressure. Also, the cocoa butter in chocolate contains some oleic acid, a heart-healthy monounsaturated fat also found in olive oil. For more from Beth Pilar and Ellen Sternau, see pages 23 and 189.

Makes about 1 cup melted chocolate

PREP TIME: 10 MINUTES + 5 MINUTES REFRIGERATION TIME

½ pound dark baking chocolate

1 tablespoon vegetable oil

24 strawberries, dried apricots, and/or pretzel rods

Melt the chocolate with the vegetable oil in the microwave. Heat it in 10-second intervals and stir in between. The oil keeps the chocolate shiny.

Dip the fruit or pretzels into the melted chocolate so that they're two-thirds covered. Place them on waxed paper and then refrigerate for 5 minutes. Serve immediately.

PER SERVING (1 CHOCOLATE-DIPPED STRAWBERRY):
30 CALORIES • 0 G PROTEIN • 4 G CARBOHYDRATES • 2.5 G FAT

Chocolate, Fig, and Almond Bites

Stored in the refrigerator, a batch of these bites will last for weeks. "They also make a great trail or running snack before, after, or during a workout," Patricia Wells says. To make them, fill paper petit-four cases (72 of them) or mini-muffin liners on a baking sheet.

Dark chocolate boosts cardiovascular health, figs are an excellent source of fiber, and almonds cut cholesterol levels when eaten as part of a low-saturated-fat diet. For more from Patricia Wells, see pages 16, 50, 104, and 194.

Makes about 72 small bites, or 60 larger bites

PREP TIME: 20 MINUTES / REFRIGERATION TIME: 30 MINUTES

$3\frac{1}{2}$ ounces bittersweet chocolate (such as Valrhona Manjari 64%), chopped

$\frac{1}{2}$ cup honey

$\frac{1}{3}$ cup hottest possible tap water

Peel of 1 lemon, grated

$\frac{1}{8}$ teaspoon fine sea salt

$\frac{3}{4}$ teaspoon ground cinnamon

1 cup dried figs, stems removed, finely chopped (about 5–6 figs)

1 cup unblanched almonds, toasted and coarsely ground

Combine the chocolate, honey, and water in a small saucepan. Heat the mixture over moderate heat just until the chocolate melts. Stir to combine. Remove from the heat. Stir in the lemon peel, salt, cinnamon, figs, and almonds.

Arrange the paper cases side by side on a baking sheet. Spoon the mixture into the paper cases, using a demitasse spoon, filling each about $\frac{3}{4}$ full (about 2 teaspoons each). Refrigerate them for at least 30 minutes to firm up before serving. The bites will keep in a sealed container for several weeks.

PER LARGER BITE: 40 CALORIES • 1 G PROTEIN • 5 G CARBOHYDRATES • 3 G FAT

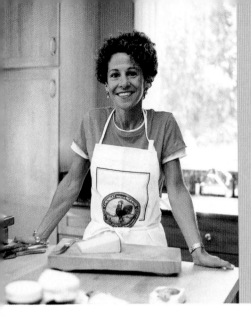

LAURA WERLIN

Laura Werlin quit her job as a broadcast journalist in San Francisco to become a writer about something she loves: cheese. The author of four books about cheese eats it for breakfast, lunch, and dinner, and hopes that her near-daily runs of 3 to 4 miles each keep her cholesterol in check. "My running is more 'slow and steady wins the race,' which means I've had no knee or hip problems after 16 years of running so far," she says. Afterward, cheese—that is, light, sweet artisanal cottage cheese—is still her choice to refuel. For more, go to laurawerlin.com.

Chocolate-Hazelnut and Goat Cheese Melt

QUICK AND EASY

This dessert, a recipe from Great Grilled Cheese, *is a simple but unusual combination of Nutella, a chocolate-hazelnut spread, and goat cheese. Serve it with coffee and sweet pear slices. "It's like a hot fudge sundae without the ice cream," Laura Werlin says.*

Makes 4 servings

PREP TIME: 10 MINUTES / COOK TIME: 5 MINUTES

8 tablespoons (about ½ cup) Nutella or other hazelnut-chocolate spread

4 ounces fresh goat cheese, at room temperature

2 tablespoons butter, at room temperature

8 slices country white bread (¼" thick)

Stir the Nutella and cheese together in a small bowl. Butter 1 side of each slice of bread. Place 4 slices on your work surface, buttered side down. Spread the cheese mixture evenly over the 4 slices so that it is about ¼" thick (any thicker and the sandwich will be too gooey). Place the remaining 4 bread slices on top, buttered side up. If you wish, you can cut off the crusts (this helps pinch the bread together to create a tight seal).

(continued on page 184)

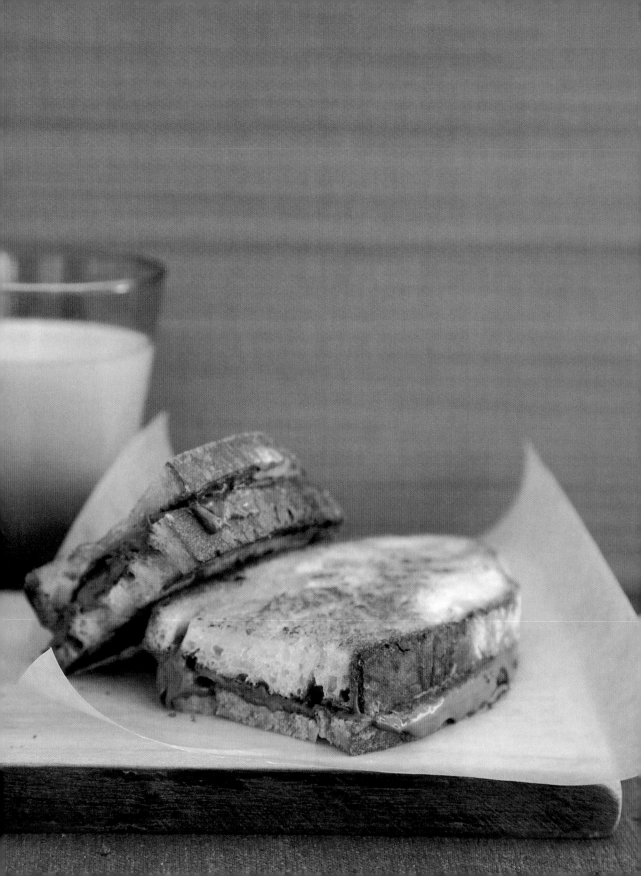

Heat a large, nonstick skillet over medium heat for 2 minutes. Put the sandwiches in the skillet, cover, and cook for 2 minutes, or until the undersides are golden-brown and the cheese has begun to soften.

Uncover and flip the sandwiches with a spatula. Cook for 1 minute, or until the undersides are golden brown. Turn the sandwiches again and cook for 30 seconds, or until the cheese is soft and creamy. Serve immediately.

PER SERVING: 560 CALORIES • 17 G PROTEIN • 63 G CARBOHYDRATES • 19 G FAT

TUESDAY EVANS

Tuesday Evans started running nearly 2 decades ago to get fit after her son was born. "Now I run so I can eat chocolate," says the pastry chef. "It helps that chocolate is the original energy bar." Besides the quick carbohydrates, chocolate—especially the dark variety—contains antioxidant flavonoids that fight high blood pressure and heart disease. Evans herself can attest to chocolate's training benefits. She started a mail-order chocolate torte business called Empire Torte a few months before she ran the 2002 Boston Marathon to raise money for charity. "While I was training, I was trying to get the recipe for my torte just right," she says, "so suffice it to say I sampled a lot."

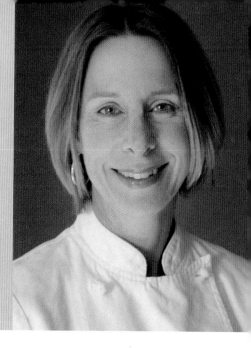

Finishing Kick Chocolate Sauce

QUICK AND EASY

This sauce for pouring over ice cream has two surprising ingredients: ground espresso beans—to give it flavor and texture—and olive oil. "It sounds weird," says Tuesday Evans, "but the oil really harmonizes with the dark chocolate." For more from Tuesday Evans, see pages 160 and 168.

Makes 4 servings

PREP TIME: 10 MINUTES / COOK TIME: 5–7 MINUTES

4½ ounces high-quality dark chocolate (60% cocoa or higher), chopped

¼ teaspoon pure vanilla extract

⅛ teaspoon caramel, orange, or raspberry flavoring (optional)

1 tablespoon extra virgin olive oil

¼ teaspoon ground espresso beans

Melt the chocolate slowly in a double boiler. Once completely melted, add the vanilla extract, flavoring (if using), olive oil, and espresso beans one at a time, stirring slowly after each to avoid air bubbles. Place a scoop of your favorite ice cream in a cone or dish. Take the pan out of the double boiler and, while resting it on the stove top, tip it a bit toward you. Quickly dip your ice-cream cone in the chocolate mixture, or use a spoon to drizzle over ice cream in a bowl. Within a few moments it will harden and form a thin shell on the ice cream.

PER SERVING: 200 CALORIES • 2 G PROTEIN • 18 G CARBOHYDRATES • 15 G FAT

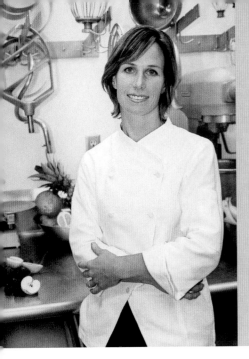

MEGAN ROMANO

Megan Romano began making and selling cakes in high school, which is also when she started running, to offset extra calories. Things haven't changed much for the chef since then. The effort Romano now puts forth in the kitchen as the executive pastry chef at Charlie Palmer Steak and Aureole, both in Las Vegas, is matched by the effort she puts into her daily workouts. Romano runs about 20 miles a week through Red Rock Canyon. She also bikes and swims, racing in sprint-distance triathlons. "Running is similar to cooking," says Romano, who is originally from Connecticut. "To run you don't need anything but your shoes, just like all you need is a knife in the kitchen." For more, go to charliepalmer.com.

Flourless Chocolate Cake

This special-occasion treat for health-conscious runners still benefits from chocolate's antioxidants. Anthocyanins have been shown to decrease inflammation and repair exercise-induced muscle damage. Dark chocolate also improves cardiovascular health by helping to reduce high blood pressure.

Makes 8 servings

PREP TIME: 25 MINUTES / BAKE TIME: 15–20 MINUTES

1/2 cup granulated sugar

8 ounces dark chocolate (sweetened) or bittersweet chocolate, coarsely chopped

4 ounces unsalted butter

5 egg yolks

5 egg whites

Preheat the oven to 350°F. Coat a 10″ nonstick baking pan with a removable bottom with cooking spray and sprinkle with 2 tablespoons of the granulated sugar.

Melt the chocolate and butter in a stainless-steel bowl over a pot of simmering water. Set aside.

Whip the egg yolks on high speed until they double in volume. Sprinkle with 1/8 cup of the granulated sugar and continue whipping for 1 minute. Set aside.

Whip the egg whites in a clean bowl until soft peaks form. Sprinkle in the remaining ¼ cup of granulated sugar and continue whipping until medium peaks form.

Gently fold the egg yolk mixture into the melted chocolate-butter mixture using a rubber spatula. Lastly, fold the egg white mixture into the chocolate-yolk mixture, folding just until incorporated without losing volume. Pour the batter into the prepared baking pan and bake for 15 to 20 minutes. To determine when the cake is finished, insert a toothpick into the center of the cake and pull it out. If the toothpick is clean, the cake is done. Allow it to cool. (The cake may deflate and crack either in the oven or afterward; both are fine and don't affect the taste.) You can top the cake with whipped cream.

PER SERVING (WITHOUT WHIPPED CREAM):
340 CALORIES • 6 G PROTEIN • 28 G CARBOHYDRATES • 27 G FAT

Madeleines

When Vincent Francoual meets with members of Team Vincent, who race and raise money for Minneapolis's Life Time Fitness Triathlon together, he makes sure to have some of these favorite cookies from childhood on hand. "They help motivate my team," he says. Madeleine tin molds can be found at Williams-Sonoma or Bed, Bath & Beyond. For more from Vincent Francoual, see pages 62 and 90.

Makes about 72 regular madeleines or 200 mini-madeleines

PREP TIME: 20 MINUTES / BAKE TIME: 5 MINUTES

½ cup granulated sugar

2½ cups flour

1 tablespoon + 1 teaspoon baking powder

Grated peel of 1 lemon

Grated peel of 1 orange

2 sticks + 6 tablespoons butter

6 eggs, whisked

1 tablespoon pure vanilla extract

Preheat the oven to 350°F. Mix the sugar, flour, and baking powder together. Mix the lemon and orange peel into the dry ingredients. In a separate bowl, melt the butter. Let it cool for a short time and then add the eggs and stir to blend. Add the butter mixture to the dry ingredients and mix well. Add the vanilla extract and mix until blended. Let it rest for 40 minutes.

Spray a madeleine tin with cooking spray and pipe the batter into each mold until half or two-thirds full (equal to about 1 tablespoon each in a regular madeleine tin; 1 teaspoon in a mini-madeleine tin; or 2 teaspoons in a mini-muffin pan). Bake at 350°F for about 5 minutes or until lightly golden around the edges. Serve with warm Chocolate Sauce and vanilla ice cream.

PER SERVING (ABOUT 2 MADELEINES, 6 MINI-MADELEINES, OR 3 MINI-MUFFINS): 120 CALORIES • 2 G PROTEIN • 10 G CARBOHYDRATES • 8 G FAT

Chocolate Sauce

Makes 1 quart

PREP TIME: 5 MINUTES / COOK TIME: 5 MINUTES

1 pound bittersweet chocolate

2 cups (1 pint) heavy cream

1 cup half-and-half

Pinch of ground red pepper

Chop the chocolate into small pieces. Bring the cream, half-and-half, and the red pepper to a boil. Pour the hot liquid on the chopped chocolate while whisking until the chocolate is melted. If not melted, place the sauce over a hot-water bath.

PER SERVING (2 TABLESPOONS): 100 CALORIES • 1 G PROTEIN • 4 G CARBOHYDRATES • 9 G FAT

BETH PILAR AND ELLEN STERNAU

Beth Pilar and Ellen Sternau collaborate on pastries, cakes, and other treats at their New York City bakery, How Sweet It Is. But when it comes to running, "we have different styles," says Sternau, who is also a personal trainer. "I like to go faster than Beth does." Both women agree that running helps alleviate the pressure that can come with operating their own business. "It's when I organize my thoughts and take stock of what I have to do that day," says Pilar. Says Sternau, "I love the way it makes me forget about everything except my goal to finish my run." For more, go to howsweetitispastry.com.

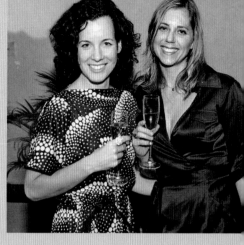

Red Velvet Cupcakes

This cupcake version of the classic Southern dessert gets it name from the reddish tinge in cocoa, which comes from the antioxidants in cocoa known as anthocyanins. The red color intensifies when the cocoa reacts with the acids in vinegar and buttermilk, but you can kick up the hue with red food coloring, too. Anthocyanins, which color other red and blue fruits and vegetables, can help reduce inflammation and counteract muscle damage from exercise. For more from Beth Pilar and Ellen Sternau, see pages 23 and 180.

Makes 24 cupcakes

PREP TIME: 25 MINUTES / BAKE TIME: 15–20 MINUTES

Cupcakes

- 1½ cups granulated sugar
- 2½ cups cake flour
- 2 tablespoons cocoa powder
- 1 teaspoon baking soda
- 1 teaspoon salt

- ½ cup vegetable oil
- 1 cup buttermilk
- 2 large eggs
- 2 tablespoons red food coloring
- 1 teaspoon pure vanilla extract
- ½ teaspoon vinegar

(continued on page 191)

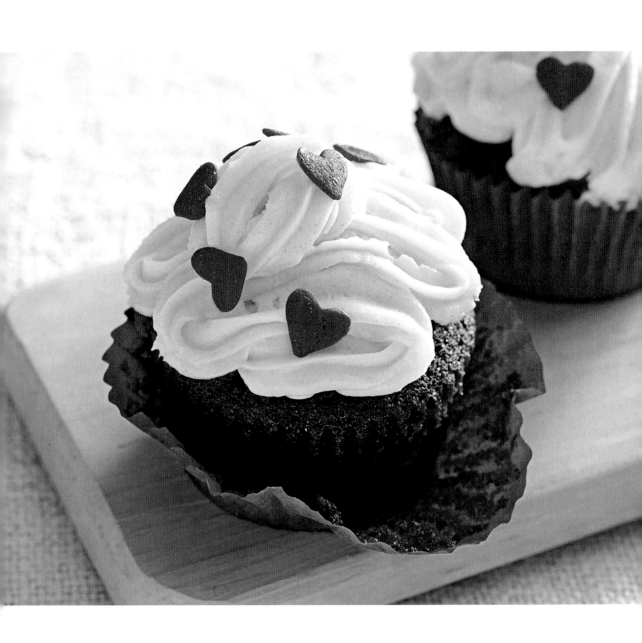

Frosting

8 ounces cream cheese (1 bar), at room temperature

½ pound (2 sticks) unsalted butter, at room temperature

2 cups confectioners' sugar

1½ teaspoons pure vanilla extract

Heart-shaped cupcake toppers or colored sugar

Cupcakes

Preheat the oven to 325°F. Line two 12-cup muffin pans with paper liners. Mix the sugar, flour, cocoa powder, baking soda, and salt together in a medium-size bowl. Mix the oil, buttermilk, eggs, food coloring, vanilla extract, and vinegar together in a separate bowl. Pour it into the dry mixture and stir until combined. Fill the muffin cups two-thirds full with batter and bake for 15 to 20 minutes, or until the cupcakes spring back from the touch. Cool in the pan on a rack for 10 to 15 minutes. Then, remove to the rack and cool completely.

Frosting

Mix the cream cheese and butter together until smooth. Slowly mix in the confectioners' sugar, then add the vanilla extract. Frost the cooled cupcakes using a piping bag fitted with a star-shaped tip, or use a small spatula. Sprinkle the cupcakes with colored sugar or use cupcake toppers.

PER SERVING: 290 CALORIES • 3 G PROTEIN • 35 G CARBOHYDRATES • 16 G FAT

Roasted Pineapple à la Mode

This 220-calorie treat is surprisingly large and buttery, Devin Alexander says. Pineapples are especially rich in the antioxidant vitamin C and manganese. One cup provides 128 percent of the Daily Value for this trace mineral, which is critical for energy production. For more from Devin Alexander, see pages 123 and 124.

Makes 4 servings

PREP TIME: 20 MINUTES / COOK TIME: 20 MINUTES

8 fresh pineapple rings (¾" thick)

2 tablespoons light butter (stick, not tub), melted

2 tablespoons light brown sugar

2 cups fat-free, double-churned vanilla ice cream

Preheat the oven to 400°F. Line a large baking sheet with parchment paper. Place the pineapple rings side by side on the prepared baking sheet. (If you have one, use a small, round cookie cutter to core the slices.)Use a pastry brush to spread half of the melted butter over the tops, and then sprinkle evenly with half of the brown sugar. Bake for 9 minutes.

Flip the rings and brush them with the remaining melted butter, and then sprinkle with the remaining brown sugar. Bake another 9 to 11 minutes, or until the pineapple is golden-brown and warmed through. Divide the rings among 4 dessert plates or bowls. Scoop ½ cup ice cream on top of each and serve immediately.

PER SERVING: 220 CALORIES • 4 G PROTEIN • 45 G CARBOHYDRATES • 4 G FAT

Strawberries with Balsamic Vinegar `RECOVERY`

Strawberries get their bright-red color from antioxidant anthocyanins that help counteract inflammation and muscle damage from exercise. One cup of strawberry halves contains just 49 calories and nearly 150 percent of the Daily Value for vitamin C—more than an orange.

In this recipe, the acidity of the vinegar brings out the sweet-tartness of fresh strawberries. Joe Bastianich advises using the highest-quality balsamic vinegar on hand. For more from Joe Bastianich, see page 95.

Makes 4 servings

PREP TIME: 5 MINUTES

¼ teaspoon balsamic vinegar

1 teaspoon sugar

1 pint clean, hulled strawberries (about 2 cups)

Add the vinegar to the sugar in a large bowl. Gently toss the strawberries into the mixture. Marinate for a few minutes and serve.

PER SERVING: 27 CALORIES • 1 G PROTEIN • 7 G CARBOHYDRATES • 0 G FAT

Watermelon-Cantaloupe Salad

"This simple salad is pretty, delicious, and light," Patricia Wells says. Watermelon is a good source of lycopene, an antioxidant that can fight cancer and heart disease. Cantaloupe provides vitamins A and C; 1 cup of cantaloupe balls contains more than 100 percent of the Daily Value for each vitamin. For more from Patricia Wells, see pages 16, 50, and 104.

Makes 4 servings

PREP TIME: 5 MINUTES

2 cups watermelon balls

2 cups cantaloupe balls

Bunch of mint leaves, rinsed and destemmed

Combine the watermelon and cantaloupe in a large bowl and dress with the mint leaves.

PER SERVING: 60 CALORIES • 2 G PROTEIN • 14 G CARBOHYDRATES • 0 G FAT

Index

Underscored page references indicate boxed text. **Boldfaced** page references indicate photographs.

Conversion Chart

These equivalents have been slightly rounded to make measuring easier.

VOLUME MEASUREMENTS

U.S.	Imperial	Metric
$\frac{1}{4}$ tsp	–	1 ml
$\frac{1}{2}$ tsp	–	2 ml
1 tsp	–	5 ml
1 Tbsp	–	15 ml
2 Tbsp (1 oz)	1 fl oz	30 ml
$\frac{1}{4}$ cup (2 oz)	2 fl oz	60 ml
$\frac{1}{3}$ cup (3 oz)	3 fl oz	80 ml
$\frac{1}{2}$ cup (4 oz)	4 fl oz	120 ml
$\frac{2}{3}$ cup (5 oz)	5 fl oz	160 ml
$\frac{3}{4}$ cup (6 oz)	6 fl oz	180 ml
1 cup (8 oz)	8 fl oz	240 ml

WEIGHT MEASUREMENTS

U.S.	Metric
1 oz	30 g
2 oz	60 g
4 oz ($\frac{1}{4}$ lb)	115 g
5 oz ($\frac{1}{3}$ lb)	145 g
6 oz	170 g
7 oz	200 g
8 oz ($\frac{1}{2}$ lb)	230 g
10 oz	285 g
12 oz ($\frac{3}{4}$ lb)	340 g
14 oz	400 g
16 oz (1 lb)	455 g
2.2 lb	1 kg

LENGTH MEASUREMENTS

U.S.	Metric
$\frac{1}{4}''$	0.6 cm
$\frac{1}{2}''$	1.25 cm
1″	2.5 cm
2″	5 cm
4″	11 cm
6″	15 cm
8″	20 cm
10″	25 cm
12″ (1′)	30 cm

PAN SIZES

U.S.	Metric
8″ cake pan	20 × 4 cm sandwich or cake tin
9″ cake pan	23 × 3.5 cm sandwich or cake tin
11″ × 7″ baking pan	28 × 18 cm baking tin
13″ × 9″ baking pan	32.5 × 23 cm baking tin
15″ × 10″ baking pan	38 × 25.5 cm baking tin (Swiss roll tin)
1$\frac{1}{2}$ qt baking dish	1.5 liter baking dish
2 qt baking dish	2 liter baking dish
2 qt rectangular baking dish	30 × 19 cm baking dish
9″ pie plate	22 × 4 or 23 × 4 cm pie plate
7″ or 8″ springform pan	18 or 20 cm springform or loose-bottom cake tin
9″ × 5″ loaf pan	23 × 13 cm or 2 lb narrow loaf tin or pâté tin

TEMPERATURES

Fahrenheit	Centigrade	Gas
140°	60°	–
160°	70°	–
180°	80°	–
225°	105°	$\frac{1}{4}$
250°	120°	$\frac{1}{2}$
275°	135°	1
300°	150°	2
325°	160°	3
350°	180°	4
375°	190°	5
400°	200°	6
425°	220°	7
450°	230°	8
475°	245°	9
500°	260°	–

RUNNER'S

→ **Everything a runner needs to know, so you can enjoy running more than ever before!**

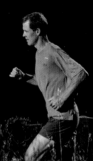

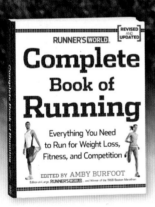

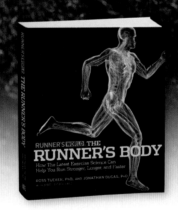

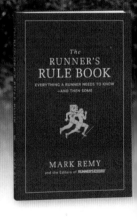

→ **Complete Book of Running**
Build strength, speed, and endurance for your best run ever! Packed with everything you need to know to run for fitness and competition and maximize your performance! Get started on the right foot!

Visit www.completebookofrunning.com/ap.

→ **The Runner's Body**
Unlock the secrets of your body and unleash your full running potential! When it comes to achieving your best on the road, track, or trail, your running can only be as good as your body.

Visit www.rwrunnersbody.com/ap.

→ **The Runner's Rule Book**
Everything you need to know about running! With *The Runner's Rule Book*, you'll discover the definitive answers to every running question you've ever asked—or never thought to ask. Get the answers now!

Visit www.runnersrulebook.com/ap.